My Awakening: Living With A Chronic Health Condition

***

Judith M.O. Brown, Ph.D., SWP

ISBN: 978-1-7347098-0-3

DEDICATION

In memory of my parents: who always championed my educational pursuits. To my mother who instilled in me the courage and tenacity that has sustained me throughout this journey. To my father who instilled in me the love of gardening and was my greatest cheerleader in my love of the arts, dancing and exploring new places. Even though you are both gone, your love continues to sustain me and give me strength.

To my dear friends, my sister from another mother, Jean, and Cousin Donna: Thank you for your continuous support, kindness, and encouragement as I continue to face the challenges of living with vasculitis.

To my doctors: I thank God for guiding you into my life. I am blessed to have such dedicated doctors and I owe my life to your skill and tremendous dedication.

To those in the vasculitis community and all those who face the daily challenges of living with a chronic health condition: Please do not let the disease define you. Continue to fight and live each day to the fullest. Treasure each day. Surround yourself with positive people, and most of all, hold onto God who knows and gives us the strength to endure. As my friend Rafael and champion always reminds me, "Giving up is not an option."

To Pat: Who stepped forward to take me to Johns Hopkins when the call came for me to receive my kidney. I treasure your love and friendship.

To my guardian angel Francesca and sister-in-Christ: You never hesitated and stepped into action when I needed you during those crucial days of hospitalization in 2018. You never left my side and I will forever be thankful for your selflessness.

PREFACE

D r. Judith Brown…a title I hold with much grace, and thankfulness, achieved after a tremendous surreal journey. Looking back, my appreciation of God's mercy and grace really began after a fateful health diagnosis in May 2006 of Anti-Neutrophilic Cytoplasmic Autoantibodies (ANCA) associated glomerulonephritis, an auto-immune disease affecting small blood vessels in the body. ANCAS target and attack a certain kind of white blood cells called neutrophils. In my case, it attacked the blood vessels in my kidney. After the diagnosis and being told it was contributing to loss of my kidney function, my initial reactions were of anxiety and frustration that my plans for completing my doctorate might be derailed, and disruption of my life goals - goals left unfinished, dreams I wanted to fulfill. However, I later learned that what I saw as a hindrance, God used as a sanctifying agent to draw me closer to him.

I chronicle this journey in the hope of inspiring and motivating others to view the diagnosis of a chronic illness not as a death sentence, or a signal to give up on fulfilling life long goals, but rather as a wake-up call to make your life count. Call it strong willed or stubbornness, I was filled with a sense of urgency, more focused on pushing forward rather than allowing my diagnosis to deter me from pursuing my goals. I refused to let my illness define me. I was determined to focus on the light at the end of the tunnel: in spite of the increasing tiredness, the endless medications, the side-effects from the medications, and my deteriorating kidney function which ultimately led to renal failure and dialysis.

I kept fighting and refused to give in to bitterness. I would not allow my circumstances to dictate my outlook and how I would face the future. As I read today's daily devotion I was reminded, "When facing a challenge, you have two choices. One is to focus on what you lack and how God doesn't appear to be responding the way you want. The other option is to recognize that your need indicates His desire to teach you something, to mold you into the person he wants you to be. Then you can rejoice over all that He plans to accomplish."

On that momentous day on October 10, 2009 when I received my transplanted kidney, I never looked back. In 2010, I ultimately gained my doctorate and was chosen as my class valedictorian speaker. It may seem like the deck is stacked against you, but looking ahead and holding unto God, He will give you the strength to overcome and succeed despite the tremendous obstacles.

FOREWORD

Congratulations Judith on such a fulfilled life. You never let the obstacles of your life from the beginning of childhood into an adult stop you from your many accomplishments. You are an amazing woman that I hope people who buy your book will be inspired by the many things you have done. Your faith in God, who gave you the vision and determination to journey the ups and downs of life has enabled you to always move forward in life – not look back. Your life has held many, many challenges that so many of us probably wouldn't have continued to persevere.

We first met working at IPMA (International Public Management Association for Human Resources) and you were taking care of your mom, who had cancer and worked full time. After the death of your mom and later your dad, there seemed to be one thing after another, but you still continued to have the faith in God that he would see you through everything. Later the kidney diagnosis was revealed and another journey began with your serious health condition.

You did dialysis at home and continued to work. Nothing stopped you --- no matter how things in life continued to get more complicated, you managed to set a path for your life that would lead you to where you are today. A successful educated woman who has worked to fulfill her goals in life.

Your many travels to other countries are another facet of your life you have been able to fulfill. You have enjoyed every place you have visited. I pray you will continue to pursue your dreams and God continues to grant you your health to do even more things.

Lots of love to you always Judith, and may God keep you in his loving care.

Pat Wood

CHAPTER 1

THE DIAGNOSIS

I t was in November 2005. I found myself feeling so tired in the mornings, even after 8 to 9 hours of sleep. Initially I chalked the tiredness up to working full-time and simultaneously pursuing my doctorate. At this time I was preparing to take my doctoral comprehensive exams. However, by December of 2005, I found that just going up the 15 flight of steps to the second level of my home was exhausting. I felt as if I was climbing Mount Everest. I have always been a very active person, so this was quite alarming. I knew that something was terribly wrong when I found myself holding unto the banister to aid my way up the stairs. To compound matters, I started experiencing pain and swelling in my shin and ankles. I did not remember hitting my shin, and wracked my brain trying to figure out when I had hit my leg.

As the days went by I felt so tired. I found myself fighting to stay awake driving to and from work. One morning I woke up after the alarm went off, and I attempted to get up as it was time to get up to get ready for work. However, I did not have the energy to get off the bed. My feet were hurting unbearably and I just did not have the energy to get up. I had to call in sick. I then called my primary care physician's office and asked if I could come in to see him sooner even though my annual visit was only one month away. I told the receptionist that I was not feeling well and it was a bit frightening.

In December 2005, I went in to see Dr. Opaigbeogu my primary care physician. I explained my symptoms and he examined me. When he took my blood pressure, he told me that it was unusually high considering it was usually in the normal range. He ordered lab-work and an x-ray of my lower leg to see if by any chance I some-how had a fracture, even though I told him that I had not been doing anything that could cause me to have a fracture. In January 2006 when the results came back a few days later it showed every-thing was in the normal range, with two excep-tions. My creatine which is linked to the kidney function was no longer in the normal range of 0.7 mg but had elevated to 2.4 mg. The lab work also revealed I had recently developed type 2 diabetes mellitus. I was stunned. Over the years, I had been pretty healthy, except for the common cold, and most recently a touch of bronchitis. These results were surprising and puzzling. Dr. Opaigbeogu wasted no time. He said he was referring me to a colleague who was a nephrologist, Dr. Buari Osman, for him to evaluate the reason for my elevated creatine levels.

At this time, my primary emotion was one of anxiety, as all that was prominent on my mind was that I did not want anything to derail fulfillment of my goals. I had so much left I wanted to do with my life: complete my doctoral degree, travel, get married, have a family. As soon as I departed his office I called and made an appointment to see Dr. Buari Osman. I was able to get an appointment for February 2006.

Looking back, I am convinced that nothing that happens or people we meet are happenstance in our lives – God has been guiding every step of my life's journey, which is why I am convinced he led me to Dr. Osman. To Dr. Osman I owe a tremendous debt, my life. It so happened that Dr. Osman suspected after my physical examination and laboratory data that my low residual renal function was not the result of diabetes as I had relatively normal renal function up until the recent diabetic diagnosis. He said he had to rule out other causes of kidney disease such as glomerulonephritis which is uncommon in an African American. He also had to rule out systemic lupus, and ordered serologic studies. He also ordered a renal ultrasound to evaluate the size and texture of my kidneys. He then advised me to measure my blood pressure readings at home to ensure it was lower than 130/80 and avoid nonsteroidal anti-inflammatory drugs while adhering to a low salt and low calorie diet.

After the serologies and all other tests did not reveal the contributory cause, he ordered a kidney biopsy to adequately define the reason for my rising creatine levels and deteriorating kidney function.

During the time I was going back and forth to my doctor appointments and getting laboratory tests done, I was still working full-time and attending my final classes in my doctoral program at Virginia Tech. It never occurred to me to take time off. I had to keep busy. Close friends kept telling me to rest, take a break from school, but if I did not remain busy then I would be spending the time worrying about what I could not control. I believe God gave me the strength so I could continue working and pursuing my studies. I had a sense of urgency to complete my doctorate, and it also served the purpose of distracting me from my health concerns.

Dr. Osman had scheduled for me to do the kidney biopsy at Southern Maryland in April of 2006. We had to wait for about two weeks for the results. It was the longest two weeks of my life.

On April 17, 2006, while at work, I received a call from Dr. Osman. He told me that my result from the biopsy had returned. He told me to go straight to Southern Maryland hospital as my creatine levels were climbing even higher and he was afraid I would go into cardiac arrest as my renal function was worsening. I think my type "A" personality kicked in or it could have been stupidity, as I began to argue with him that I had work to finish at the office and could not possibly go to the hospital now. I did not feel that sick. Dr. Osman calmly informed me that he was faxing over an order to my supervisor (I was still working full-time) for me to go to the hospital. My supervisor assured me that the work would still be there waiting and to please leave as the doctor ordered.

I felt like I was on autopilot as I drove home, got a few toiletries, and drove to Southern Maryland hospital where Dr. Osman said a room was already prepared. The nurses were already awaiting my arrival when I entered admissions. I was admitted and taken to my room. A nurse came by and I was hooked up to an IV. Later Dr. Osman came by and explained what was happening. The biopsy findings confirmed his suspicions. The pathology results revealed I had Vasculitis, which is a group of uncommon ANCA-associated (AAV) glomerulonephritis diseases, which result in inflammation of the blood vessels. AAV can affect different blood vessels in the body leading to the damage of critical organs such as the heart, lungs, kidneys, nervous system, gastrointestinal system, skin, etc. In my case, it affected my kidneys. The actual cause of these vasculitis diseases is usually not known. However, immune system abnormality and inflammation of blood vessels are common features. The kidney is the most commonly affected vital organ in ANCA-associated vasculitis. My creatine levels which were an indicator of my kidney function were climbing. He needed to begin treatment immediately to stabilize and prevent the rapid climb of my creatine functions. The treatment of renal vasculitis involves the use of a high dose glucocorticosteroids in combination with cyclophosphamide (a chemotherapy drug) to induce remission of the disease. He explained I was being given this intravenously to quickly stabilize my condition, and then thereafter would be switched to the oral chemotherapy form of the drug - Cytoxan and the oral steroid prednisone. I felt like I was in a nightmare. I only wanted to go home and tend to my garden. I kept telling myself this could not be happening to me.

Dr. Opaigbeogu who had referred me to Dr. Osman came to visit me during my hospital stay. He admitted that after Dr. Osman told him of my diagnosis he had to research it as he was unaware of the condition. That night I thanked God again for leading me to Dr. Osman and prayed he would be able to get me well. When a few days passed I relentlessly pressed Dr. Osman to let me go home. He explained he could not until my numbers were stabilized. My potassium levels were too high, which if left untreated could lead to cardiac arrest. I told him my blood pressure would normalize if I was in my own bed. He laughed and told me soon. I finally was released after my levels were stabilized and was so relieved to be going home. I had been in the hospital for a week.

There was one snag. Hospital policy dictated that I could not drive myself home, but my car was out in the parking lot as I had driven myself to the hospital and I had no other means of going home. I did not want to trouble any of my friends, and actually had not told anyone I was going to the hospital. I made up my mind that I would drive myself home. After the nurse came with my discharge orders, I never made her the wiser. I waited until the attendant came to my room. When he inquired if my ride was here to take me home, I pointed to my car which was clearly visible from the hospital window and persuaded him that I lived a short ride from the hospital. I would take the back roads and drive slowly. He was very reluctant, but I told him no one was available to take me home and it was safe as I was not going to be in traffic. He finally relented and wheeled me to my car. Yay, victory! I proceeded to drive home, window down and music loudly playing to keep me awake, praying all the way, glad to be finally going home. Looking back, now, I laugh at how brazen I was to leave the hospital on my own. I doubt if I would take that chance today but desperate times are a cause for desperate measures, I told myself.

Shortly after being home and resting comfortably in my own bed, I received a call from Johns Hopkins. Dr. Osman had referred me to the Vasculitis specialists at Hopkins for further assessment and evaluation. He explained to me that they had the best specialists to treat my vasculitis condition.

I made the appointment, and in late April 2006 for the first time met Dr. Geetha, who was later to become not only my doctor but along with Dr. Osman my champion, and voice of reason over the years as I navigated the ups and downs of my disease. She had my biopsy results sent to her and her team for further diagnosis. She confirmed I had ANCA associated vasculitis which manifested as glomerulonephritis, with rapidly progressive acute renal failure. She also made a strange remark…. that I was "lucky" – Lucky! I looked at her astonished, but she explained that it could have been worse as vasculitis can also attack other organs such as the heart, lung, or brain. I could be feeling much sicker, not able to work.

She cautioned me to keep stress to a minimum as it could exacerbate my condition. I chuckled and told her that would be a difficult task unless I moved to a mountain top. She smiled but insisted that it was important that I try. Driving home after that first meeting, I was more hopeful that all was not lost. With the diagnosis of my kidney disease, at least she explained that I could go on dialysis in the event I went into renal failure until I received a kidney transplant.

The John Hopkins team continued my treatment of Cytoxan and Prednisone until the summer of 2006. By that time, I had only 20% kidney function remaining and my doctors at John Hopkins and Dr. Osman continued to monitor my condition. Despite my doctors telling me that my kidney function could possibly deteriorate even further if the treatment did not work, I deluded myself into thinking that might not happen. I was always so health conscious, so I told myself this could not happen.

Life on Cytoxan and Prednisone
While on Cytoxan and the high dosage of prednisone my outward appearance changed. I developed the infamous moon face which is one of the side effects of prednisone: when on high doses of prednisone for an extended period of time it can cause swelling in the cheeks and in the neck. It

can also cause weight gain. Knowing the moon face was inevitable; I was determined to minimize the weight gain. I remained active which helped minimize gaining excessive weight, and did yoga exercises at home to maintain my strength and flexibility. I only gained around 5-7 pounds. The change in my appearance made me feel unattractive and was upsetting, not to mention the mood swings and insomnia. When I was at work, co-workers would stare and then quickly look away. However, I never stopped going into the office. Work kept me distracted from my illness as well as working on my doctorate. At night I would take a warm bath and drink chamomile tea so I could relax and get some sleep, even if was not a full night's sleep. The David Letterman show and gadget advertisements became my companions on many nights. The Cytoxan on the other hand caused me to be nauseous and also changed my appearance. I noticed my skin became darker and my nails became discolored. I drank ginger tea to combat the nausea. I could not do anything about the skin changes.

CHAPTER 2

MY BUCKET LIST
BEGINS - IRELAND

After that momentous meeting with Dr. Geetha at Johns Hopkins, an alarm went off. I suddenly realized that my rigid approach to life had to cease. This diagnosis was a wake-up call. Before my diagnosis, everything had to follow a certain order. Complete my education, meet the man of my dreams, get married, start a family. Getting this sick was not in my plans, but now I realized that life does not always go as we plan. I thought I needed to be married to travel to the places of my dreams. I had travelled to some parts of Europe as part of my work, but never thought of venturing to the places on my dream list on my own. I wanted to wait for marriage to travel with my husband. That kind of thinking had to stop I told myself. Who knows when or if I would meet that special someone. After my diagnosis I realized life was too short. I also had just finished reading "Eat, Pray, Love by Elizabeth Gilbert--which celebrated the writer's irresistible, candid, and eloquent account of her pursuit of what she really wanted out of life. I said to myself--why wait until getting a death sentence to start living instead of existing—so, my bucket list began. I had always wanted to go to Ireland. Chalk it up to fulfilling a childhood fantasy of finding the leprechaun and the pot of gold at the end of the rainbow... I was determined to find out...Lol. My former supervisor and now dear friend Sandra had told me about her trip to Ireland, so I proceeded to ask her for the contact information of the agent who had arranged her trip. I reached out to the agent and made arrangements. I initially made arrangements to go on my own but since I was only recently diagnosed Dr. Geetha was concerned about me travelling alone. I was determined, so she recommended I have a friend accompany me in the event I got sick on the trip. I relented.

I thought of Peg. We had become fast friends while working at my first job when I migrated to the States in 1990. She would invite me to go on trips when she would visit her family for family reunions. When my mother became ill, sometimes on weekends she would come and get me while my mom was in day care, so I could get a breather for a couple of hours. She was excited about sharing my adventure, but then remembered she did not have a passport. I checked online and saw that she could get one expedited. The week following St. Patrick's Day we were on our way! "You need to learn how to select your thoughts just the same way you select your clothes every day. This is a power you can cultivate. If you want to control things in your life so bad, work on the mind. That's the only thing you should be trying to control." - Elizabeth Gilbert, Eat, Pray, Love.

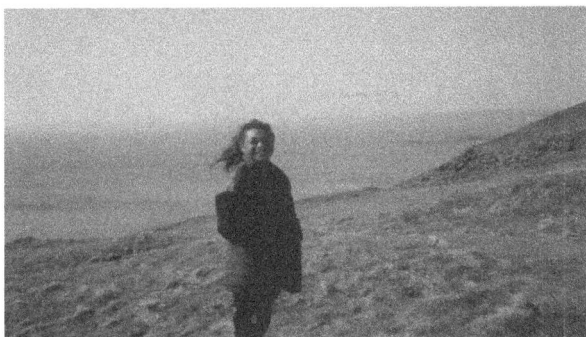

At Cliffs of Moher, Ireland: April 2007

Those 10 days in Ireland were extraordinary and mystical. Every day was better than the first. The kind and genuine warm nature of the people, the Ring of Kerry, the quaint town Killarney, the villages, the rugged cliffs, the small villages, visiting the castles and, of course my luxurious stay at Adare Manor was magical and intoxicating.. Listening to Irish songs, eating fish and chips in the Irish pubs, drinking Irish coffee, and singing on the tour bus with my new found friends was wonderful. The peat bogs and picturesque mountain ranges and the stunning scenery were even better than I pictured it. I even kissed the Blarney Stone! Another dream achieved: I actually climbed the 120 steps to get to the top of Blarney Castle and then proceeded to lean backwards over the edge while holding on to the iron bars of the surrounding wall with the help of one of the Castle attendants. In Dublin, I visited the statue of Molly Malone in the square…. Molly Malone of Dublin's Fair City…selling her "Cockles and Mussels…." To see her was to love, her," indeed… I cried when it was time to return to the States. I felt so at home there in Ireland. It was magical. I have vowed someday to return. I did not find that pot of gold, but I did find my leprechaun, who sits forever on my key ring.

On the last leg of the trip, while walking with the tour group through Dublin I found myself out of breath and unable to walk further. I told Peg to go ahead with the group and I slowly walked back to the bus, but did not tell Peg how I was feeling. I prayed I would be able to make it to the end of the trip, and I did. I got my last wind and was able to enjoy the rest of the trip.

While at the airport on our way back to Maryland I was feeling weak and could not stop shivering. I did not let Peg know how badly I felt, but I asked her if she would drive herself home and

I slowly drove back to my home praying I would make it home okay.

I was relieved to return home safely. I took my medications and slept. I felt I was coming down with a cold. I told Dr. Osman when I went for my follow-up visit. I had conducted medical labs the week before my visit, but the results showed my renal function was relatively stable. I was actually mildly anemic due to endometrial bleeding which explained my weakness at the end of my Ireland trip. He told me to continue taking my medications and he requested a repeat renal function study.

I returned to see Dr. Osman in July 2007 and he indicated that my latest renal labs showed my renal function was progressively deteriorating. I also had evidence of hyperparathyroidism, so he added another medication to my growing repertoire. He also decided it was time to educate me on the possibility of a renal transplant, and told me I was a candidate for peritoneal dialysis pending a kidney transplant. Why peritoneal dialysis? I told him I was not prepared to do Hemodialysis where I would have to spend at least 4-5 hours, 3 times as day at a dialysis center. I was still working full-time and led a busy life, attending school in the evenings pursuing my doctoral studies. I also wanted to be able to pursue my love of travel and Dr. Osman knowing my personality by now explained that peritoneal dialysis would offer me more of that flexibility. The only drawback was that I would need to do my dialysis 3-4 times every day, even while at work. Due to my small stature, I would only need to spend approximately half an hour to do the manual exchange required per session. He said once the filtration rate of my kidney dropped below 15ml per minute, I would need to have a peritoneal catheter placed in my abdomen. I pushed that thought out of my mind as I was convinced things would not come to this. I felt I would be able to beat this. I was continuing to do yoga to build up my strength and working with the nutritionist at Johns Hopkins who gave me tips on the best foods to eat for someone with kidney disease. She gave me a cookbook for those who had kidney disease: my favorite recipe was making blueberry pancakes from scratch, as it did not have artificial ingredients found in store bought pancakes. I would take the pancakes to work and my co-workers would beg me to share, saying they tasted much better than when made with store bought pancakes. It so happened that when Dr. Opaigbeogu was investigating the reason for my sudden illness he told me to stay away from all processed foods and foods with any chemicals. The nutritionist at Johns Hopkins said the same when she gave me the recipe book. The food actually tasted better and I shared so many recipes from that book with co-workers and friends. To this day, even post-transplant, I still stick to this way of eating, which is much healthier.

My doctoral courses kept me busy the next few months. Keeping busy I think saved me. I was distracted from spending a lot of my time feeling sorry for myself and remained focused on my goals. Even more importantly I also found that my relationship with God had changed. It was now more personal. I would talk to him as I would to any of my friends, crying out to him in anger when the reality of my situation hit me; talking to him when I felt alone....which was pretty often. Friends empathized, but it is funny when going through a crisis, only a few stand by you. My mother had passed away ten years before. She who would have been there by my side as my comforter and cheerleader was now gone. God became more real to me. Even though I had become a Christian as a teenager and attended church services, I really had not developed a relationship with God until my diagnosis, and my subsequent journey with vasculitis. He became my constant companion when the despondency descended and the business of work and school could not block it out.

I continued on the medication regimen prescribed by Dr. Geetha and the Johns Hopkins Renal team. Near the end of July, Dr. Geetha and her team asked if I wanted to enroll in the

Rituximab ANCA-Associated Vasculitis (RAVE) trial study for those with severe ANCA-associated vasculitis. The reason for the trial was that Cyclophosphamide and glucocorticoids had been the cornerstone of remission-induction therapy for severe antineutrophil cytoplasmic antibody (ANCA) –associated vasculitis for 40 years. Uncontrolled studies suggested that another drug rituximab was effective and may be safer than the cyclophosphamide-based regimen that was more toxic. I agreed to participate in the study, as I felt that I would be contributing to a very important cause. In addition, Dr. Geetha also enrolled me on the cadaveric transplant waiting list as no one had yet come forward to be a living donor. If my renal function deteriorated further I would need to be on peritoneal dialysis. The earlier I was on the list, the more points I would be able to earn and lessen my wait time as much as possible for a new kidney. I met with the Johns Hopkins transplant team, which included a renal transplant social worker who conducted a psychosocial evaluation. Her job was to ensure I had the resources I needed during my transplant wait, which included obtaining Medicare assistance to help finance my dialysis and the caregiver support I would need post-transplant. I convinced her that I had the support of my church and close friends who would serve as my caregivers even though I lived alone.

During this period of travail I found out a profound phrase from my childhood Church minister in Jamaica resonated…"Circumstances will reveal the true man." It sure did. When I was diagnosed it required at first being on the treatment regimen of chemotherapy and high doses of prednisone. I told Mike (not his real name) my boyfriend at the time about my diagnosis, and he was sympathetic at first, but I after a while he started making excuses, saying the drive from Virginia to Maryland, a 35 minute drive which was never an issue when I was well, had now become an issue. Even though I had not gained a lot of weight due to strict regimen of yoga and eating the right foods, I developed what is called 'moon face' a side effect of the prednisone. He said visiting me was now taking a toll on his car. There were too many potholes, and he was becoming so busy with work. I look back now and laugh at the absurdity.

During the RAVE trial I was frequently required to journey to Johns Hopkins for intravenous treatment on the trial drug on a weekly basis. Initially, the doctors required that I be accompanied by someone on my visits as they did not know how I would react to the intravenous trial medication. I told Mike but he never offered to take me. When I asked him, he kept saying he was busy with work and if it was only on a weekend. As if the clinic was going to open on a Saturday for his convenience. He had the nerve to ask me where my family was, as "he did not sign up for this." I had already explained to him the situation with my family: that we were not close knit, and I felt my heart drop as I realized he really did not care for me. What bothered me even more was that even though he never accompanied me, he also never asked how the treatment was going, or if there was anything he could do to help. I had been living the pretense of a relationship. I told him that even if I had family living in the basement, as my significant other, did he not think he should be more supportive? I decided not to argue with him, even though his indifference was painful. My mother's voice was echoing in my mind. When I used to lament to her that my close friends were all getting married and life was just passing me by, she made a comment which I now can appreciate, "Do be careful, not to be in a such hurry, that you end up picking s--it". It is best to wait to find someone who will be good for you, even if it is later on in life."

I just told Mike that God would work things out for me. My friend Peg offered and took time off from work to accompany me for a couple of the earlier visits. I was so thankful. However, I did not want her to continue taking time off from work, so I asked Sister Parker a sister from my church, if she could to take me on subsequent visits, which she was happy to do.

After the first few weeks of treatment, when I noticed I was not having an adverse reaction to the intravenous medication, I decided to drive the one hour and a half drive to and from Johns Hopkins on my own. I wanted to give Sister Parker a break, and did not want to trouble any of my friends to make that long drive. It was okay; I told my doctor and the nurses who were concerned. I had my smelling salts and told the nurses that the copious amounts of green tea I asked them to give me would keep me alert on the drive home. They found that so amusing.

On one of my follow-up visits with Dr.Geetha during the RAVE trial she commented that all was looking good except for my blood pressure which was elevated. She said it was important that my blood pressure be stable as elevated levels would only serve to exacerbate my condition. She asked if there was anything bothering me and I told there was, but I would take care of it. On the drive home I called Mike's number, but got his voicemail. I decided to leave a message. I basically told him that it made no sense pretending that all was well. If he could not be supportive during this challenging time in my life, and only wanted to be there during the good times, then it was best we went our separate ways, as life does not work like that. There is never a guarantee that one of us would never get sick or that there will never be bad times, but when you cared about someone you want to be there for them. I told him it was best we ended things as when I did not have a boyfriend; at least that was the reality. Knowing I was in a relationship and felt more alone than ever was too painful to bear. Later on that evening he returned my call. Albeit to say he did not attempt to talk me out of my decision. He actually seemed relieved I made the decision for him, and took him off the hook. Surprisingly, that night I slept better than I had in a long time. I think deep in my heart I knew things were over even before I got sick. I had just avoided the signals. As a result of my illness, God revealed the truth to me. Circumstances had indeed revealed the man.

During the summer of 2007, I continued working full-time, going to final classes and preparing my prospectus for my dissertation. As I said above, I had gained weight being on the high dosages of prednisone. However, a positive did arise; when I started treatment and during the RAVE trial my hair actually started growing. I was happy that the Cyclophosphamide and the prednisone had not caused my hair to fall out, even though I had gained weight. That was a bright spot I needed in my life. When I looked in the mirror all I could see was the dreaded "moon face" which occurs as a result of being on high dosages of prednisone. The medications had changed my appearance.

Nevertheless, I never let that deter me. I never stopped going into the office unless I had a medical appointment. I kept going to the office as work kept me occupied and distracted from focusing on my situation.

In 2007, I reconnected with a former associate, and dear friend, Rafael. We had lost touch over the years since meeting at a human resources conference in 2003. He had become a professional mentor but when we met again by chance in 2007 and I told him of my diagnosis, he became a tower of strength when I wanted to give up and I am ever thankful for his friendship and gentleness. They say God sends you angels on earth when you are in greatest need, and I believe it to be true. He supported me throughout my challenging journey, admonishing me whenever I started feeling sorry for myself and became a rock when I was at the breaking point. I remember one day sitting by the bathtub washing my hair when suddenly large clumps of my lovely hair came out in my hands. I was devastated. This was the first time since my diagnosis in 2006 that I remember breaking down and cried. It was at that moment that my world came crashing down. My hair had been growing and was the longest it had ever been despite my diagnosis and this had given me so much hope. Losing my hair was a great blow to my spirit. Rafael said the most important thing for was for me to get better. My hair was falling out but I needed to focus on the end result – getting better. "Your hair will grow back." When I started developing the dreaded moon face from the prednisone, and started to gain weight and could no longer fit into my clothes, he wisely said that gaining weight was better than the alternative, death. "You still are beautiful." He always knew how to keep me laughing and feel better about my situation. He never indulged my self-pity, but always showed me that things could be worse. I will never forget one day we were having lunch and I threw up. I felt so ashamed and kept apologizing, but he shushed me and made light of it asking if I was pregnant. Yeah, Immaculate Conception, I retorted and we both laughed.

In October 2007 on my 18 month visit to Johns Hopkins, Dr. Geetha indicated my labs revealed my condition was stable and they considered me to be in remission. She said they would cease administering the RAVE medications which I was now receiving in pill format and not intravenously. I was now at stage V chronic kidney status, and I told her that I would consider going on peritoneal dialysis as Dr. Osman had advised when the need arose, until I received a transplant. I was to continue my monthly blood work so they could closely monitor my kidney function and my vasculitis. I was also to continue administering Procrit, a medication I self-injected weekly to maintain my red blood cell count at a normal level. Without it I would be severely anemic.

By this time, Dr. Geetha had already placed me on the cadaveric transplant waiting list and I had already met with the Johns Hopkins transplant team. Over the years prior to my transplant, the team became a tremendous source of encouragement and support. Every month I had to do blood work and send in samples to the Johns Hopkins team so they could have my antibody status in the event a cadaveric kidney became available for matching. My assigned transplant specialist was supportive and became an e-mail life line, sharing jokes that would uplift my day and words of encouragement when I had to be on dialysis.

By September 2007, I was going for three month follow-up visits to John Hopkins since I was now considered in remission. I was forging ahead and busy working on my dissertation prospectus with the hope of defending in the spring of 2008. I was excited and anxious at the same time, but thinking good thoughts.

My birthday celebration in October was quite enjoyable. I took the day off from work for my birthday that Friday and went to my favorite Spa in Waldorf for a deep tissue massage. Since I was diagnosed in 2006, I had made a promise to myself to not wait for a gift card to get a massage or pamper myself. The diagnosis was a wake-up call for me to take the time to pamper myself on a regular basis and not consider it a luxury. That Sunday, my former boss and close friend Sandra prepared a lovely birthday brunch for me. Jean a former colleague and close friend was also there. We three had a ball and afterwards went strolling through the wonderful Brookside Gardens near Sandra's house. That was the great highlight of my birthday celebration. I forgot my illness that weekend.

It continued to be busy at work coupled with the fact that I was working on my prospectus. I had planned to go to New Jersey to be with a former college friend and her family but I was so tired, I stayed home and rested.

A few days after Thanksgiving, Pat a dear friend sent me an email story which I am convinced involved God's hand. It was titled ---Never give up."

One day I decided to quit... I quit my job, my relationship, my spirituality...
I wanted to quit my life. So, I went to the woods to have one last talk with God.

God", I asked, "Can you give me one good reason not to quit?"
His answer surprised me...: "Look around", He said. "Do you see the fern and the bamboo?"

"Yes", I replied.

"When I planted the fern and the bamboo seeds, I took very good
care of them. I gave them light, I gave them water. The fern quickly
grew from the earth. Its brilliant green covered the floor. Yet nothing
came from the bamboo seed. But I did not quit on the bamboo.
In the second year the fern grew more vibrant and plentiful. And again,
nothing came from the bamboo seed. But I did not quit on the bamboo.

He said. "In year three there was still nothing from the bamboo seed.
But I would not quit. In year four, again, there was nothing from the
bamboo seed. I would not quit." He said. "Then in the fifth year a
tiny sprout emerged from the earth. Compared to the fern it was
seemingly small and insignificant...But just 6 months later the bamboo
rose to over 100 feet tall. It had spent the five years growing roots.
Those roots made it strong and gave it what it needed to survive. I

would not give any of my creations a challenge it could not handle."

He asked me. "Did you know, my child, that all this time you have been

struggling, you have actually been growing roots". "I would not quit on

the bamboo. I will never quit on you." "Don't compare yourself to

others." He said. "The bamboo had a different purpose than the fern. Yet

they both make the forest beautiful." "Your time will come", God said to

me. "You will rise high"

"How high should I rise?" - I asked.

"How high will the bamboo rise?" - He asked in return.

"As high as it can?" - I questioned.

"Yes." He said, "Give me glory by rising as high as you can."

God was sending me a reminder that He was watching over me. It came at the very time I needed a lift.

In January of 2008 I developed a cold which I tried to treat by taking home remedies. My condition prevented me from taking over the counter medications which would elevate my blood pressure. However, my home remedies failed to make me feel better. In addition I felt tired and run down. I went to my primary care physician Dr. Opaigbeogu who diagnosed I had bronchitis. He prescribed antibiotics to help clear up the infection and bed rest for a week.

I had my follow-up appointment with Dr. Osman in February. My blood pressure levels had become elevated as a result of my bronchitis and my January lab work indicated my white cell and red blood cell count had fallen. In reviewing the lab work with me, he said it showed my renal function was slowly deteriorating. He increased my blood pressure dosage and told me to resume my weekly injections of Procrit to increase my hemoglobin (i.e. my red cell count).

CHAPTER 3

PERITONEAL DIALYSIS

B y the spring of 2008, I was still feeling fatigued. Each morning I would ask God to give me the strength to arise from my bed and get ready for work. It was getting more difficult to get out of bed, even after 8 hours of sleep. I had a follow-up appointment to see Dr. Osman on May 6th.

I decided not to go into work that day, as I was feeling so tired and weak. Dr. Osman did not have good news. My April labs revealed my kidney filtrate rate had fallen to 11 ml per minute. He said I was experiencing progressive renal function deterioration and suspected my extreme fatigue was due to abnormally high levels of waste products in my blood. I also had Stage 1 hypertension. He increased my blood pressure medication and told me to monitor my blood pressure readings at home for any further adjustment in my medications. He ordered repeat renal function lab work to see if the filtrate rate continued to be less than 15 ml per minute. If it was, he would recommend placement of a peritoneal dialysis catheter for initiation of dialysis. I tried to argue with him that I was preparing to defend my prospectus and could I delay this. He stated firmly that the delay of renal replacement therapy would only lead to further complications. He also advised I follow up with the Johns Hopkins transplant center for preemptive kidney transplantation, if feasible. Based on my last meeting with the transplant team, they had said with my common blood type, O positive, it would be an approximate 4 to 6 years wait time before I would receive a cadaver kidney. My heart sank and anxiety set in as I feared my prospectus defense could be derailed.

My repeat renal function labs revealed my filtration rate had again dropped below 15 ml per minute. It was decided. Dr. Osman referred me to the Washington Hospital Center team to conduct the procedure to insert the catheter. I met on May 19th with the surgeon who was to conduct the procedure at the Hospital for him to examine me and go over the procedure. My dear friend Pat had offered to accompany me. He examined me and I did preoperative procedures. The pre-op revealed all was well and he scheduled the surgery for May 30th.

I had my prospectus defense scheduled for that summer, and had been making edits to the chapters as my professor reviewed them. Dr. Osman said the dialysis would help while I waited for a kidney to become available. I prayed for strength to get me through what was going to be a challenging journey.

I know God was with me every step of the way. He provided a support system of not only good friends, but the transplant team also became a source of hope. One member of the team who I will call Audrey, when I told her I was going to need to be on dialysis uttered the comforting words my mother always said to give me courage. "Please try to keep your chin up." She encouraged me to take heart in the fact that peritoneal dialysis would allow me more freedom that hemodialysis would. She promised me when I asked God to give me the grace to navigate this transition in my life, HE would and that gave me comfort.

On May 30th, I was having the catheter inserted in my abdomen at Washington Hospital Center. As I was being prepped for surgery, the surgeon came over and told me Dr. Osman called to check to see if I had made it for surgery. I had to laugh. Dr. Osman did not trust that I would have showed up considering how I had argued with him about putting it off with my upcoming prospectus defense. He knew how I could get, always questioning things. If he recommended any change in medication I would question him to death about its benefits and then tell him I was going to investigate it on the internet. When he told me my kidney function had deteriorated further and I needed to be on dialysis I knew he was right, but I was frightened. Even though I was reluctant, I knew I had to face reality. I believed him when he said if I did not go through with the dialysis to improve my filtration rate, I would not be defending anything. I was determined to be well. The surgery was an outpatient procedure. When I woke up after the surgery, I had to almost strangle the nurse in the recovery room who kept going back and forth, even when I kept calling him as the pain ripped through me. After what seemed an eternity, he finally gave me some morphine. Pat who had accompanied me, took me home that evening, and stayed overnight to ensure I was okay. At first I did not want to bother her to stay, but she and Rafael convinced me it was best she stayed in the event I needed assistance having just had surgery. Looking back I am ever so thankful for the wonderful friends with which God blessed me.

They had given me Percocet to take for the pain after the surgery. However, I only took it for a few days before I switched to Tylenol as I did not like how it made me feel. After a few days, in June, the nurse at the dialysis center near me changed the dressing and went over the dialysis expectations with me. I started training the following week after the surgery on how to execute the peritoneal dialysis exchange on my own. When I looked at the area where they inserted the tube near my navel, my first thought was that I looked like an alien with this tube sticking out of me. After my first day of training, I sat in the parking lot of the dialysis center and broke down. It suddenly hit me that this was going to be my life for a while. The transplant team had said that the wait for a cadaver kidney for someone with my common blood type of O positive would be a 4 to 6 year wait. What man would want me with this tube hanging out of me and having to do dialysis every day? That evening Rafael spoke words of encouragement and reminded me of my blessings, telling me I was a strong woman. I so needed to hear that. I started dialysis the week of the 24th after I was healed from the surgery.

God had been good to me so I tried not to spend my time worrying. My mother used to say to me, "When you pray, let it go. Let God take over." I could not waste needed energy worrying. Work was still busy and kept me going. I also was consumed with working on my prospectus as my defense was scheduled for July 24th. That gave me time to prepare for the presentation and also get oriented to doing dialysis. Doing dialysis daily took its toll emotionally at times, but I asked God for strength each day and to be thankful for his mercy. I tried to make the best of it and live each day the best I could.

Initially, I started doing the dialysis manually 3 times a day, every day: in the morning when I woke up, at lunch time at my office and at bed time. It became my routine. When my close friend Rita in Las Vegas emailed me to check-up on me I actually made a joke of it. So far, I told her I was trying to do the best I could to get the hang of it, however it was a good thing I wasn't the socialite as my social life would be in the doghouse. My other indulgence was my garden. I now found more time to "stop and smell the roses." I found gardening quite therapeutic and always found a new specimen to add to it.

I decided to also make arrangements to go to Jamaica that August after completing my defense. My dialysis nurse assured me that many of her patients travelled even while on dialysis. There was one couple she said who went on a cruise every year. It just meant making arrangements with the DaVita dialysis group to have my dialysis supplies shipped to where I was staying, for example my hotel. I so desperately wanted to be back in familiar Jamaica, when I was healthy and full of life. I was looking forward to getting some ocean breeze, swim in the ocean and hang out with old friends. I planned on squeezing every drop of pleasure out of that.

In July, two days before my defense Dr. Osman referred me to see the Director of the Transplantation services at Washington Hospital

Center for evaluation to get on the transplant list in the Washington DC and Virginia area. This he said would increase my chances of getting a cadaver kidney. At the time, I was only on the Johns Hopkins waiting list for the Maryland area. The Director was very pleasant and kind. He was concerned that no relatives had stepped forward to donate the kidney, but I assured him I was keeping my faith that God would prevail in getting me a kidney even if it was to be a cadaver. My vasculitis was in remission and I was off the immunosuppressants. The issue was that a live donor kidney would be better than a cadaver as it would last longer. He was pleasantly surprised I was defending my prospectus in only a few days, with all that I was going through. He suggested I also consider going on the waiting list at a Midwestern transplant program if possible as in the Midwest the ratio of patients waiting to donors is more favorable than in the Washington metro area and my waiting time would be much shorter. He was hoping that a living donor would occur for me. He added me to the Washington Hospital waiting list, but said it was likely that it would be a number of years before a standard criteria donor became available. He conceded that a deceased donor or pediatric kidney would also be okay for me to receive, so waitlisted me for those categories.

July 24th – Prospectus Defense Day!

The day of my prospectus defense, July 24th dawned. I was a little nervous but so ready to share my dissertation topic with my committee. All went well with the Defense. Hooray!! My committee was thrilled with my presentation. They said the Prospectus is one of the best they read and were looking forward to my survey results! God had really been guiding me through these hurdles. My defense was initially scheduled for June, but one of the committee members could not make that date, so it was moved to July, This was great for me as it gave me time to recoup and get acclimatized to being on dialysis. God worked things out perfectly.

In late July, my peritoneal dialysis nurse said I could graduate to using the dialysis machine. My spirits lifted, as this meant I would no longer need to do manual exchanges with the bags 3 times a day, but would do my exchanges throughout the night with the dialysis machine on my night stand, and only one manual exchange at lunch time at the office. I was excited about using the machine instead of always doing the manual exchanges. The downside was that at night I would have had tubes running from my abdomen to the machine and also to my bath tub to empty the toxin waste. I jokingly said to my friend Rita that maybe it was a good thing I was not married, as my husband would be tripping over the tubes at night. I also found trying to fit into some of my clothes with an abdomen full of dialysis fluid a little challenging. The blessing was that the fashion trends at the time were baby doll tops and empire waist dresses, which meant my looser fitting clothes, did not appear out of place. I tried to carry on as best as I could. The dialysis helped to give me back some of the energy I had lost due to the deterioration in my kidney function. I did not realize how tired I had become with the vasculitis condition until I felt the difference with being on peritoneal dialysis. When I went in for my checkups at the dialysis clinic, I saw and heard from other patients who had to do hemodialysis that it made them so tired. Strange as it may seem, I felt so blessed to be able to do peritoneal dialysis. Do not get me wrong, since my diagnosis with glomerulonephritis, there were days I was so despondent thinking my life was a living nightmare, wondering if I had to live like this for the next 4 to 6 years before I could receive a new kidney. However, as challenging as it was having to do peritoneal dialysis, with 3-4 exchanges a day, the plus side was that it afforded me the flexibility and independence to do it in the comfort of my home, or when on travel. I even continued to work full-time. I did not have to resolve myself to lie on a bed in a dialysis center 3 days a week for 4-5 hours doing hemodialysis.

As hard as it was, I had to seek out the positives of my situation in order to continue on this journey. I literally had to pinch myself at times to snap out of the negative thoughts when they descended. I would also think about my mother during those times. I was determined to keep positive and "keep my chin up" as my mother used to encourage me whenever I felt down.

CHAPTER 4

ESCAPE TO JAMAICA

After the successful defense of my dissertation prospectus, it was time to plan my trip to Jamaica or "Jamdown" as my friends and I refer to our childhood hometown!! God had been by my side the entire time that day. I did not feel nervous once the committee members started posing questions about my proposed research. I came through with flying colors, as they gave me the blessing to pursue my investigation. I was so happy that hurdle was behind me. I could now focus on sending out my survey. However, my trip to Jamaica was all I could think about. I so needed that break.

I was scheduled to depart for Jamaica on August 22nd for a week. The peritoneal nurse assisted me in getting in contact with the DaVita authorities to arrange for my dialysis supplies to be shipped down to Jamaica. I was scheduled to stay at the all-inclusive Spanish RIU resort in Ocho Rios highly recommended by a friend. I was tingling with the anticipation.

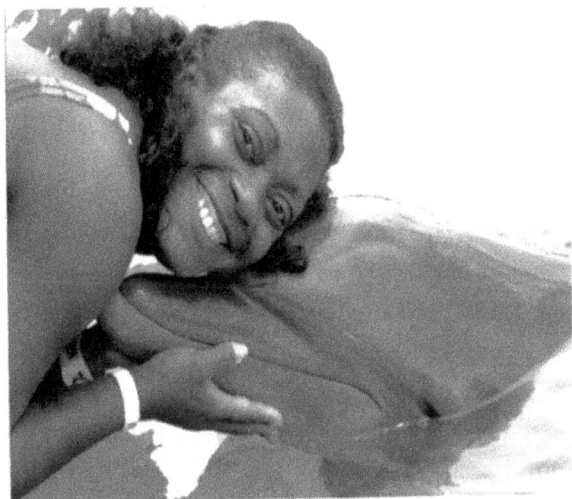

Jamaica – Swimming with the Dolphins- August, 2008

I had made arrangements with the hotel manager weeks before my arrival. I spoke to the manager about my medical situation and the need to have a driver pick me up at the airport and accompany me to the cargo area to retrieve my dialysis boxes. The manager kindly recommended I use one of their private drivers, rather than attempt to take a regular taxi. The medical company was shipping 5 boxes down to Jamaica. Initially I thought they would be shipping it directly to the hotel, but I was told, they had to go through customs so that was not feasible. The hotel manager was another one of the angels God sent me. She assured me that a driver would be there to pick me up and assist me in retrieving the boxes. I could now relax and look forward to my visit.

I arrived in Jamaica at Sangster's International Airport in Montego Bay on August 22nd 2008. After exiting the luggage claim area to the to the transport area, I stood there looking around and it suddenly hit me that I did not know how to recognize the driver. I had no clue and had forgotten to ask the hotel manager. However, as soon as I went outside, this gentleman approached me and asked me if I was Ms. Brown. That was a relief. He figured it was me since I was looking around as if looking for someone, and he took a chance I was looking for him. I told him about the boxes and he said he would pull up the van he had driven since the manager had told him about me retrieving the boxes from customs. That was a trial. Thank goodness he was the right man for the job. Without him I would have been unable to navigate the intricate process of filling out paper work at one office then going back and forth in the hot sun to one office then another. Finally he asked me if I had any money to "assist" with accelerating the process. I only had US dollars so he advanced me some Jamaican dollars to use to "move" the process along and we were able to retrieve my boxes very quickly after that. God was indeed working.

My stay at the RIU was awesome! Looking back, I realize that it was what I needed most. The previous two years since my diagnosis, continuing to work fulltime, and diligently working on my prospectus, I needed that break to breathe, forget the negatives and just take care of me. It was no accident when I arrived that while waiting for them to get my room ready due to an oversight, and frustrated as my dialysis exchange was overdue, I was told that I could do my exchange in the nurses' quarters nearby. The driver put one of my boxes in the office and I went in. When I explained to the nurse what I needed to do, she instantly smiled and said she was actually a former dialysis nurse and was familiar with peritoneal dialysis. If that was not God, I do not know what is. That was too much of coincidence that the resort I chose to stay on my visit had a nurse who had experience working with dialysis patients. My heart sang. She mentioned how expensive it was for Jamaican patients who needed to do dialysis and I offered to leave any unopened bags with her as a donation to the hospital or any clinics. She was very thankful.

During my one week stay, I had great Jamaican food and the staff was courteous and wonderful. Every day I would walk to the beach and relax on a beach chair, read and people watch. I scheduled to go the recent famous attraction at the time, Dolphin Cove. That was a wonderful adventure. I went walking on the jungle trails, interacting with exotic birds, snakes and iguanas. I even held an iguana and took a picture with him! I also went kayaking and swam with the dolphins. I had no time to feel despondent, but enjoyed every moment of my trip.

Tina, a former high school friend, came to visit me at the resort. It was great seeing her again after so many years. The last time we had seen each other was at my father's funeral in 1999 when six months after my mother died, I had to go down to make arrangements for his burial and service. "A true friend is someone who reaches out for your hand and touches your Heart." God indeed blessed me with dear friends. During that period when my mother, then father died, close friends stood by me, helping me over the tough terrain. Now, when I was going through this tough period of needing a kidney, their moral support was buoying. She took me to dinner at a popular jerk chicken eatery nearby, where we ate, talked, laughed and reminisced about old times.

There was a threat of a hurricane coming towards Jamaica in the final few days of my stay – Hurricane Gustav. The hotel staff boarded up the glass front of the hotel where we had meals. It was predicted that where we were on the North Coast, we would not be hit hard, but we had heavy lashing rains. We had no problems at the resort. The last two days, Thursday the 28th and Friday the 29th it rained and we lost power for only a short time. I was out taking pictures with the rest of the tourists that Friday. Saturday morning dawned and the sun came back out. Barry the driver came and got me early so we could tour Ocho Rios before my flight that afternoon. He bought me a dozen "Juici" Patties to take with me, and also gave me two CD's with reggae singer Tania Stevens' songs. He had been playing her songs in his car whenever he would drive me around and I commented that I liked her. He was surprised I had not heard of her and said I had been out of touch for too long. During the hurricane, while hunkered down at home, he had made copies of her songs on CD's for me. He was a very kind man. Another angel God put in my path.

**Return to the States
– Transition to Dialysis Machine & Shingles**
Upon my return to the states, I was as busy as a bee. I disseminated my survey to my two sample groups and resumed my full-time work schedule. One friend emailed and asked if Stella was back! When I was preparing to go down to Jamaica to get rejuvenated, she said in Jamaican patois, "Yes mi dear Stella. Go get yu groove back!!" I had a real belly laugh at that. I emailed her back, "Yes, my dear, Stella is back at the grindstone." I admitted to her that doing the dialysis and taking all the medications got a bit depressing at times, but

I tried to snap out of it as best I could. I tried to look for the silver lining whenever I could in my situation. In September, I was given the green light by my dialysis nurse that I qualified to transition over to using the dialysis machine at night. I would now be reduced to doing only one manual exchange at my lunch break at work, and at bed-time hooked to the machine, I would be able to do continuous dialysis exchanges while sleeping. The nurse trained me on how to use the machine. She and I laughed when I told her, my love life was really going to be non-existent with me being hooked to a machine at night with the tube from my stomach hooked to the machine and the other tube from the machine running across my bed into the bathtub to empty the fluid contents. Nonetheless, I was so relieved, as this was so much better than doing 3 manual exchanges every day. I could now attend after-work activities and accept social invitations in the afternoon without having to make excuses to leave early and rush home to do an exchange. Instead of accepting the invitations and departing early, I just turned them down.

One day my church minister called me. I had been included on the church's prayer list since my diagnosis in 2006. One of the church sisters' had approached him as she wanted to offer to be living kidney donor for me. I was so overwhelmed as I had resigned myself to waiting the 4- 6 years that the transplant team and the "number of years" the specialist at Washington Hospital Center had predicted I would have to wait on the deceased donor waiting list. I gave him the necessary contact information to reach out to the Johns Hopkins Transplant coordinator and waited. I asked him if the church sister was absolutely sure she wanted to do this for a stranger. Did she have the necessary support system (i.e. family) to aid her during and after the surgery if she proved to be a match? He said he and his wife would be willing to help her with whatever support she needed during the recovery, as she lived alone. I waited. One day the church sister called me at home, quite upset. She had gone in for her evaluation and had undergone the rigorous screening process that a living donor has to undergo to determine not only physical but mental fitness to be a donor. Unfortunately they discovered she had medical issues that even though not critical at that time in her life, would greatly affect her later on in life. She was disqualified. Ironically, I found myself consoling her. She protested that she was only occasionally having medical issues. I told her the doctors knew best, as they had better knowledge of her condition and to be a donor there had to be no question that you did not have a potentially debilitating condition. Not only could she be at risk, but as the transplant recipient I also could be harmed by her health condition.

Chin-up, I told myself. I took comfort in the fact that a stranger was willing to step forward and donate her kidney. No one else had offered. I was not angry, but allowed myself the time to grieve before I snapped out of it. God was in control. I asked Him for the comfort to endure. I was still on the waitlist, even though my wait would be 4 to 6 years. Most importantly, I was still able to get up in the mornings, albeit how tired I was, get ready and drive to work. With my dissertation defense behind me, my focus was now on the survey investigation. I was so immersed in keeping busy, I could not stay depressed for too long. God gave me the strength to continue.

October dawned and also my birthday. Peg and I went out to Linden, Virginia on our annual road trip to the Apple House to get their delicious Alpenglow sparkling cider made right there in Linden and their other apple treats - apple fritters and apple cider and apple butter donuts to die for. Not to mention their specialty sauces; and of course my favorite spice, SLAP YA' MAMA. To round off a truly wonderful weekend I had dinner that Sunday with my two great friends, Sandra and Jean.

November came around, and my monthly check-up. I was rejoicing and giving thanks that day after the doctor reported my labs were looking good. Surprising, a few years before having good labs was not something I would rejoice over. Each day, despite the challenges of fatigue, I tried to find the silver lining. That Thanksgiving in 2008 I gave thanks for my doctors, friends and most of all to God for giving me the strength to endure.

In February 2009, I received an e-mail from Mary, a childhood friend from Jamaica who lived in Canada. I had not heard from her in years. It was Friday and I was at work but it was a beautiful day. It was my break and I was actually doing some school work. It was my final year!!!!! I had a bad week with some challenges with my dialysis and was trying to psyche myself out. At times I felt so despondent when I thought of spending the rest of my days on dialysis. I would read the Psalms to get some comfort from David. I would read the bible when I did not feel up to talking to God, but at other times, HE was the only one I could talk to as humans did not always understand.

The quote at the end of Mary's e-mail signature gave me comfort, especially with the feelings of despondency I had been experiencing.

His quiet streams of peace are deep,
We've yet to drink our fill, by half;
And we, the Master's trusting sheep,
Find comfort in his guiding staff.

–Randal Matheny

In early March, 2009, I developed a burning, tingling, itching pain along the right side of my body, including the right side of my face. After a few days I developed a group of fluid-filled blisters that were red and inflamed on the right side of my face. I immediately contacted the office of my dermatologist and made an appointment to see her. When she saw me, she immediately diagnosed I had shingles. As a child, I had contracted the virus Chicken Pox, and with my compromised immune system she said the virus was awakened. She was also concerned how close it was to my eye, and said it could potentially cause infection in the cornea, so she ordered me to see my ophthalmologist immediately after leaving her office. She gave me a prescription for an antiviral medication – Valtrex to help the sores heal faster, keep new sores from forming, and to help decrease the pain and terrible itching. I called my ophthalmologist's office after leaving the dermatologist and explained the situation. The receptionist told me to come in. When I saw the doctor, I told him that I had shingles and just came straight from the dermatologist. He could see how close the rashes were to my eyes. He wrote a prescription for antibiotic eye drops for me to take a few times a day for a couple weeks and then follow-up with him. I stayed at home for about two weeks to recuperate and recover from the bout of shingles. It was a miserable two weeks.

The pain subsided after the first week, thank goodness but I kept looking in the mirror to see how well the medication was working to reduce the rashes.

I emailed the transplant coordinator on March 10th to let her know that I would not be able to do my monthly blood draw to test my antibodies which I did the 10th of every month because I had contracted the shingles. My dialysis nurse was planning to draw my blood the following Friday after I was no longer contagious. The coordinator replied that it was okay to send in the sample late as If there was a significant change in my antibody status, the lab needed to know.

It was St. Patrick's Day and my follow-up with my ophthalmologist. I was all decked out in my green and having reminiscent thoughts about my trip to Ireland. He was pleased with my progress. The infection was clearing up nicely in my right eye. With my immune system so compromised, these unpredictable episodes with infections could arise he said. He wanted me to continue the drops for another week. I continued to be vigilant and prayed that I would have no more dramatic episodes. I returned to work after St. Patrick's Day. The worst was over, and I was feeling better. I continued working on my dissertation analysis. I needed to have my final analysis completed by July 2009, so I took a week of leave from work to write at home in peace during the Easter week. It was less stressful. I could not wait for the dissertation process to be over. I decided I would take occasional breaks until I did my defense so I would not be as stressed with the work at the office.

CHAPTER 5

STOP AND TELL GOD THANK YOU
NEW ORLEANS AND CADAVER
CALLS BEGIN

After the Easter week, I received an email from my friend Rohan in Jamaica. It was quite timely. I was weary from the waiting and being on dialysis, As much as I tried to keep busy, it would rear its ugly head. In these times, God found a way to remind me that he was by my side.

Dear God,
I want to thank you for what you have already done.
I am not going to wait until I see results or receive rewards; I am thanking you right now. I am not going to wait until I feel better or things look better; I am thanking you right now. I am not going to wait until people say they are sorry or until they stop talking about me; I am thanking you right now. I am not going to wait until the pain in my body disappears; I am thanking you right now. I am not going to wait until my financial situation improves; I am going to

53

thank you right now. I am not going to wait until the children are asleep and the house is quiet; I am going to thank you right now. I am not going to wait until I get promoted at work or until I get the job; I am going to thank you right now. I am not going to wait until I understand every experience in my life that has caused me pain or grief; I am thanking you right now. I am not going to wait until the journey gets easier or the challenges are removed;

I am thanking you right now. I am thanking you because I am alive. I am thanking you because I made it through the day's difficulties. I am thanking you because I have walked around the obstacles.

I am thanking you because I have the ability and the opportunity to do more and do better.

I am thanking you because FATHER, You haven't given up on me. God is just so good, and He's Good all the time.

I thanked Rohan for sending that timely email and for his thoughtfulness.

I had registered to go to a professional conference in New Orleans hosted by my professional association, SHRM, near the end of June and I was excited and so looking forward to having the nice break. In May I made the necessary arrangements with DaVita to send my dialysis supplies to the hotel I was staying in New Orleans.

The economic downturn in 2009 was taking its toll. Living with a chronic health condition can be costly. I was deeply thankful to God for giving me the strength to still be able to work full time so I could maintain my health insurance. Even then I had to apply for supplemental Medicare to cover my dialysis medical expenses. I had to be so careful with my budget. Who would have thought that in the short space of a year, the economy would have declined so much that it affected the housing market. I thanked God he had given me the resources to keep afloat. I got tired a lot more easily, even with the dialysis, so tried to pace myself best I could. Dr. Osman had also prescribed Renvela for me to take twice daily due to high levels of phosphorous in my system. This was common for those who are on dialysis. I so looked forward to the weekends and the three day holiday weekends so I could remain at home to rest and work on my dissertation. I was busy as a bee working on my final chapter to send off to my advisor by July for my defense in the fall of 2009. I was tired, but pressing on.

My trip to New Orleans was looming. I was scheduled to stay at the Hampton Suites near the French Quarters. I heard the rooms were very nice and I was right across the Conference Center where the SHRM conference was being held. I could just walk across the street.

My dialysis supplies had been shipped to the hotel, and when I checked in I asked the manager to have the boxes taken up to my room. I had a

3M hook which I took with me whenever I travelled since being on dialysis. I hung it on the wall next to a chair so I could do my dialysis exchange. I chuckled to myself as I realized that the hotel staff at the hotels I stayed when I travelled must have been dying with curiosity and speculating on the reasons a guest would hang a 3M hook in their hotel room.

Staying at a hotel across the street from the conference center was a godsend. I had to do the exchanges three times a day, so I did one when I woke up in the morning before heading over to my first session, then went over to the hotel at lunch time to do another exchange before heading out to lunch. I linked up with Nadine, a former co-worker who I still kept in touch with on LinkedIn. We had arranged to link up when we found out we were both attending the same conference. We had a grand time in our free time, exploring and taking in the city.

The food was excellent as my friend Sandra who was from New Orleans had described. When I told her I was going to New Orleans she gave me tips on the places to go and where to get the best food. I ate beignets and had coffee at the Café Du Monde. The Mulate restaurant had great and delicious food, but no alligator for me even though on the menu. I enjoyed Gumbo and ate shrimp po boy sandwiches during that week at the conference.

I even had a virgin Mint Julep. I went strolling one night along the famous Bourbon Street with Nadine and some other ladies who were attending the conference. We took in the music, and people watched as people in all manner of dress danced in the streets. We even did a bit of karaoke, which was an unforgettable highlight. I got a little tired after walking for a bit, and lagged behind the others, but I totally enjoyed myself that night.

After the conference was over, I had a free day before heading back home. I arranged to tour the French Quarters via the mule carriage ride, which was awesome. I learned so much as the knowledgeable guide spouted a fountain of information that covered the storied history of New Orleans, discussing everything from their resilient culture to the aging but beautiful architecture. It reminded me so much of Europe which I love. I also did a tour of Oak Alley, a former sugar plantation, which is a national landmark and well preserved. It was like being taken back in time. The tour was very educational and called for sober reflection, knowing the plantation relied on enslaved men, women and children. It was quite an experience.

First Cadaver Kidney Call

On my return to Maryland and over the July 4th weekend John Hopkins called. They indicated they had a kidney that may be a potential match.

They cautioned me not to eat anything as they ran a battery of tests to determine if I was a potential match. I was a bundle of nerves and could not sleep as they had called late at night. I had to wait about 8 hours. Finally early in the morning the coordinator called back and said there were two other people who were ahead of me on the wait-list, so they received the kidneys. I was tired and disappointed and called the coordinator of my transplant team to explain how the process really worked. I was so confused. She explained that they normally called those who were potential matches and if the persons before me were not available I would have been the recipient. I now had to be on the alert for future calls as it was obvious I was close to the top of the list. I alerted Pat who had volunteered to take me to Johns Hopkins when I received the call to receive a kidney. I guessed God had given me a trial run so I would know what to expect when it was my turn. There is no time for preparation unlike when you get a kidney from a living donor. You had to be ready to go when they found a close match. I had sleepless nights thereafter wondering what other preparation I needed to make, but I asked God to continue to guide and watch over me. When I told Rafael about the first call he suggested I have a hospital bag ready with toiletries, a nightgown, a dress gown, underwear, slippers, something to read, and of course my charged cell phone. He taught me how to text as I had no idea how to text. When I saw Dr. Osman on my next clinic visit he was so optimistic and said it was a very good sign having gotten this first call, as that meant I should expect to get more calls moving forward. I was now on tender hooks, wondering when the next call would come.

Early August arrived. I had become a bit anemic as my hemoglobin became low and I was getting very tired. Dr. Osman had to increase my Procrit injection dose to increase my red blood count. I was so close to completing Chapter 5 of my dissertation and planned to send it off to my advisor by the end of the week to review.

Second Cadaver Kidney Call

On August 7th, I received a call from the coordinator at Johns Hopkins. I called Pat to be on standby, while I again waited, full of anxiety and again a bundle of nerves. I also e-mailed Rafael. I tried to text him but was making too many errors. The nurse called back. I sat down. Another blow, the pathologist doing the biopsy found cancer cells in the donor kidney. There was no need to run further tests. For some reason I was not despondent. I was disappointed but Dr. Osman's voice rang in my head. I would continue to get calls until the right kidney came along. He had given me the screening questions to ask when I got the calls. What was the health of the person who died? What was the age of the person? How did they die? What was their creatine level at the time of death? He emphasized I did not have to accept a kidney just because one became available. I could refuse if I did not feel comfortable with their answers. I should aim to get the healthiest one available. I told Rafael in the e-mail what the nurse said and that I would not give up hope. My bag was packed, as he had instructed me. The third time maybe the charm. I thanked him for his support. It meant so much. Onward I told myself.

Third Cadaver Kidney Call
The Labor Day weekend and Saturday, September 5th 2009 started out as normal day. I ran my errands, did my dialysis exchange then headed out for a girls evening get together with Jean and Sandra over at Sandra's house. Sandra had invited us to a girls' night together at her home with Jean and was going to make me virgin 'Mint Julep' in honor of my trip to New Orleans that summer. I was on my way when my cell phone rang. The nurse coordinator said there was a possibility a kidney may become available as there was an accident and the person may not make it and was a kidney donor. I told her I was on the way to a get together over a friend's house and should I return home instead of going. She said to go to my friend's house and as it

might take my mind off things while I waited to hear back from her. I gave her Sandra's number as well. When I arrived at the house Jean was already there. I told them both about the call, but told them it did not sit well with me that I was waiting to hear that someone died so I could get a kidney. Even though I was waiting to receive a cadaver kidney, actually waiting for someone on life support to die was a bit unsettling, to say the least. We prayed instead that he would pull through, and that the right one would come along. We decided to not focus on the situation and enjoy the evening. We had a great time, eating the lovely meal Sandra prepared. I had brought her a pie for her belated August birthday, which we had for dessert and while she and Jean had the "real" drinks (gin and tonic), I was happy drinking my virgin mint julep she had prepared for me. Halfway through the evening, her phone rang. It was the nurse. She apologized to me and said that the accident victim's loved ones refused to take him off life support. I quickly told her it was okay. I was relieved. I thanked her and said next time, hopefully it might be the right one. I told Sandra and Jean, and even though disappointed, they agreed with me that my time would come. God was in control. It was becoming so exhausting to go into work each day. I did not have much leave time, so I only took an extra day off after the holiday and

returned to work the Wednesday after Labor Day.
I was now near the top of the waitlist for the transplant so I was very optimistic and driven, despite
the weariness. I told myself God was in control
and should not waste needed energy worrying.

The week after Labor Day my advisor e-mailed
me her edits to Chapter 5 of my dissertation, so I
was kept busy and my mind occupied making the
corrections. Sandra emailed me to check-up on me
and to see if I had received any more "calls" from
the transplant team. I laughingly told her that I
had not yet received any calls since that last drama
at her house. I told her I was so thankful I was not
alone that evening, but was with her and Jean. I
had a great evening in spite of the ordeal with that
call. I promised to keep her posted when the next
call came. She responded that she hoped the next
call will be "THE ONE" and I would be able to
have a "real" mint julep!

I received an email from a former high school
classmate in Jamaica in late September. She was
quite depressed that her life was not going the
way she wanted, and seeing her siblings making
strides and progressing ahead of her professionally.
Amazingly, I found I could find the strength to
console her, even though I had my own struggles.
I let her know that in keeping the faith, she could
find her way with God's guidance. I could now
speak from experience to let her know that He

would take her through the storm, even though she was at her lowest point.

October arrived and I remained busy with work and going back and forth making edits to my dissertation submitted by my advisor and members of my committee. It kept me from sinking into depression. I was trying to make the dialysis work for me as best I could, taking one day at a time. It was becoming so expensive so I decided to apply for supplemental Medicare to help with the costs.

On October 7th I had to go for an appointment at Johns Hopkins, and per usual they took vials of blood, in this instance 15 vials not only for my regular kidney check-in but also for the study in which I was enrolled. Dr. Geetha was pleased that I was doing relatively well with no major illnesses. My vasculitis was still in remission and there was no evidence of a flare-up. When conducting my physical exam, she did note I had developed an umbilical hernia, a result of the volume of my dialysate. She recommended I discuss lowering the volume with Dr. Osman. I was to continue with my prescribed medications, taking my Procrit injection for my hemoglobin and glucose medication as needed. I was also to do my lab work every 2 months so she could continue to track my progress. I was to return to the clinic in 4 months' time.

I actually went back to work after the two hour drive from Johns Hopkins after the appointment. I felt I had been run over by a truck, I was so tired, but I guess I wanted to prove to my boss that I would not "slack" off from with so many medical appointments. The funny thing is that I was entitled to take leave under the Family Medical Leave Act for a serious health condition but back then I was more concerned with the perception of me being out of office. Looking back I do not know why I felt I had to prove myself so much at work, that I would jeopardize my health. Even though I still have a type "A" personality, I no longer put work above my health. My vasculitis diagnosis was an awakening that there is more to life than a 9-5 job. I realized later that I had to have more of a balance in my life. I wanted to make it count by doing more of the things that I was passionate about.

CHAPTER 6

THE FINAL CALL - THE GIFT OF LIFE

Friday, October 9th arrived, the start of another 3 day weekend; Columbus Day holiday weekend. Cam my co-worker and friend sent me an email reminding me of the fact that I may just get another call this weekend as two of the previous calls had occurred over a holiday weekend and this was my birthday month. Thinking back on the last three calls, I was not enthusiastic about reliving the anxiety and disappointment. When I did not respond, she came by my office and seeing my dejected persona, with her usual cheerful self told me to buckle-up. "Always stay positive. This might be it! This may be your last day in the office for a while." I could not help but smile at her enthusiasm I told her I would try. My hospital bag was packed and I was planning on getting my hair done and baking an apple walnut pudding that weekend.

Saturday came and I did my usual morning yoga workout session with my favorite wellness Channel known at that time as "Veria Living." I ate breakfast and did my household chores. I planned to fix soup after my hair appointment. I showered then headed out to my hair appointment. While doing my hair, my hairdresser and I chatted. She asked how I was doing and how much longer did I think I had to wait. I told her I had been getting calls but they had not worked out. However, I was trying to stay positive. She enquired about the process for someone to donate and I told her I would send her the information when I got home. I told her I was so looking forward to the holiday. I had plans to make an apple walnut bread pudding for the first time and was excited.

After the appointment I remembered I needed another ingredient for the soup I was making for dinner, so I headed out to the market. I was almost there when my cell phone rang. It was a nurse coordinator from Johns Hopkins. She said they had a kidney for me. I was very apprehensive. I told her I was on my way home to fix something to eat as I had not eaten since morning and she replied, great. We need you to have an empty stomach. I then asked if she was sure, as I had been disappointed three times now. She laughed and said, 'yep'! The doctor said this one has your name on it. I proceeded to ask her the questions Dr. Osman had told me to ask: How did the person die? How old were they? What was their health status? What was their creatine level? My donor who had died in an accident was thirty-eight years old and a male. He had been healthy prior to the accident. With my heart beating fast, I quickly told her yes, I would accept. God is this it?! I asked as I spun my car around in the parking area of the Miller Farms market store. On my way home I quickly dialed Pat's home number. Her husband Joe answered and I told him that the hospital called and said they had a kidney. It was real this time and I needed her to come and get me. He said she had just walked in the door. She had been at a wedding. I had called just in time. God's timing was perfect. She told him to let me know she was going to change and leave out right away. Joe said it would take about 30 minutes for her to arrive. They lived in Washington DC. At home, I quickly checked to see if I had everything ready in my hospital bag. I packed the charger for my cell phone, and then waited anxiously for Pat to arrive. It was the fall season, so even though it was only after 5:00 pm, it was almost dusk when she arrived. She asked if I had the address and then helped me lock up. We were then on our way. As we were driving I texted Rafael that I received another call and this time Pat and I were on our way to the hospital. Pat said she would follow-up and call him to give him updates.

When we got to downtown Baltimore, Pat realized she was unsure how to get to the Comprehensive Transplant Center. It was now really dark outside. She stopped and went into a gas station to ask the attendant for direction. He came outside and showed her which street to turn on. We were not far away. Thank God! Upon arrival, we went to the admission area. It was so funny when we got there; I was basically skipping when we got to the reception area. The nurse at admission actually asked which one of us was the patient. When I said me, she was surprised. She said most patients don't look as healthy as I did, and I laughed. I was so thinking back to earlier that day when I did my morning yoga workout and then went to the hairdresser. God was preparing me for this moment.

After admission, I was taken to my room. The doctors told Pat it was going to be long night so it was best she went home and they would call her. They had to do further tests prior the surgery. They proceeded to take a sample of my blood in order to be cleared for surgery: once a potential donor is identified, you need to do another test to make sure that your antibodies will not attack the donor's organ. This is done by mixing a small amount of your blood with the donor's blood. The test showed no antibody reaction. I had what is called a "negative crossmatch." This meant the transplant could proceed. The transplant could not be done if my blood formed antibodies in response to the donor's blood.

The attendant wheeled me to the surgical room. Outside the operating room, the attendant stopped the stretcher and helped me walk into the operating room where I was helped unto the operating table. After inserting my IV and putting on my oxygen mask, the anesthesiologist told me to take deep breaths, and then I was out.

Waking Up

Before my kidney failure, I had paid no attention to how important they are. When operating correctly they remove toxins from the blood via the urine and return the cleansed blood back into the body. They also regulate the levels of water, salts, acids and different minerals the body needs for good health. They even produce hormones that regulate blood pressure, glucose, hemoglobin and other body functions. After surgery I was admitted to the intensive care unit (ICU). The nurses told me the surgery went well, and the doctors were pleased my new kidney had started working immediately as noted by the urine output in my catheter bag. Kidneys donated by family members usually start working more quickly than those from unrelated or deceased donors. Yes, God's hand was at work!

The attending nurse explained that I would remain in ICU for the next 24 hours so they could ensure my vitals were stable and my new kidney was working well. Thereafter, I would then be transferred to the transplant unit. If I experienced pain at the surgical site I could squeeze the pump connected to my IV which allowed me to self-administer the morphine at set times. I was not experiencing a lot of pain but I was extremely hungry. I was not experiencing nausea which sometimes occurs after surgery. I had not eaten since early Saturday morning. She laughed and said I could only have chicken broth as I was still in intensive care. I smiled and told her I obviously took after my mom. After she had surgery and woke up in intensive care she told me she was hungry. They gave me broth to give her, but she was still hungry and asked for something more. I could only give her apple sauce and told her the same thing the nurse was telling me. She was not happy. She had me laughing. The nurse laughed again and brought me a second cup of broth after I finished the first cup in a couple of gulps and told her I was still hungry.

I was admitted to the transplant unit the next day where I would remain for two weeks. The transplant doctor came to see me. He checked my incision area. He explained that the procedure had gone smoothly. My new kidney was placed in its new home in my right lower abdomen, below a 7" incision. During transplantation, my old kidneys were not removed. That only occurs if the old kidneys are diseased. So now I had three kidneys! They were going to continue to monitor my vitals. My creatine level was continuing to lower so that was a good sign and all my other vitals were stable. My dialysis catheter was however still in place. He explained that I would return to the surgeon at Washington Hospital Center to have this removed after they determined the new kidney was fully functional and there would be no need for further dialysis.

I was still in some pain, but it was mainly a dull ache that was really only painful to the touch or when I made the wrong movement. I was taken off the pain medication administered by the IV and was taking codeine as needed and extra strength Tylenol as needed.

Pat came to see me and told me she had called Rafael and my Aunt Hazel to let them know I had the transplant and it was successful.

My Aunt Hazel, my mom's older sister who is now deceased, lived in New York. She was so thrilled when she called my room. She used to check up on me every weekend when I was diagnosed in 2006. When my mother passed away we had become very close and she had become like a second mom to me over the years. She was now a lot more confined at home with health issues so could not travel as she used to in the past. She was so worried when I was diagnosed with vasculitis and had subsequent kidney failure. She was so happy I could now live a more normal life. She said she would call my older brother Junior who lives in Minnesota and my cousin Donna who lives in Canada but to whom I was very close. Rafael sent a fruit basket since I was not allowed to have any live plants or flowers for a few weeks, and was on a strict schedule of immunosuppressants at high dosages to prevent rejection of my new kidney. This weakened my immune system and put me at high risk of infection from the bacteria in live potted plants and the water in flowered vases. He was on business travel, so he called me almost every evening to see how I was progressing.

As the days went by, I spent the time catching up on my reading and watching television. Since working on my doctorate I had no free time to do any leisure time reading, or watch shows, so I used the time while I was there to play catch-up on movies and my reading. Each morning the staff would draw my blood to check how well my kidney was functioning and all other levels. The results showed my creatine level was falling, indicating the new kidney was functioning well. Then when I thought I would be going home soon, my transplant surgeon came and told me that my lab work was showing my white cell count was rising and my creatine levels had also begun to climb. My transplant doctors ran checks to see if I had developed an infection. I became anxious. When Rafael called that evening, I conveyed what was happening and that my creatine level was rising again. He reassured me to stay positive and to keep fighting. Talking to him that evening lifted my spirits. The doctors could not find evidence of an infection after running several tests. There was only one option left. Do a biopsy of the kidney to determine if it was failing. There was potential risk of bleeding but I agreed to do the biopsy to determine if the transplanted kidney was being rejected.

The biopsy was successful and when the results came back, there was no indication of rejection. The doctors then realized that it was the trauma of the surgery which had elevated my white cell count. As it started to fall, my creatine levels also began to fall. The nurses weighed me every day, and I noticed I was losing weight. The physical therapist came by and encouraged me to walk. They needed to know I could walk on my own when I returned home. She accompanied me on my first walk around the hallway and a short flight of stairs since I told her I had stairs at home. Each day I would walk two laps around the hall-way. When I looked in the mirror, I noticed my face and cheeks had more color. I so wanted to go home. I did not want to spend my birthday in the hospital. With my creatine level now stabilized and the new kidney functioning, the doctors finally said it was okay for me to go home. I had been in the hospital for 2 weeks. I was delighted. It was Friday, October 23rd, three days before my birthday!

I called Pat with the good news. After she arrived and I had my discharge orders, I was on my way. I had a follow-up appointment scheduled at the Transplant clinic one week after my discharge. Ever since Rafael's large fruit basket had arrived, I had given an apple or orange or two to the staff who came to my room. On my way out the staff was waiting outside to wish me bon voyage. I laughed and told one of the nurses to please enjoy the rest of the fruit. I had taken a couple of the apples to take home.

Once home, I was so happy to get into my own bed. Per discharge instructions, I was to resume normal activity as I could tolerate. I could resume driving after 4-6 weeks and was not allowed any heavy lifting or strenuous activity. I was to also wear sunscreen of SPF 30 or greater when out in sun as a transplant recipient, as the transplant medications increase the risk of skin cancer. I would be on immunosuppressant medication for life, but it was a price I was willing to take if it meant not being on dialysis and living a more normal life. I was also prescribed additional drugs to reduce the risk of infection for the first month post surgery. The urethral stent and my PD dialysis catheter were to be removed in another month.

My diet was carbohydrate controlled and I could continue to have lots of fruits and vegetables, and no red meat. I could also now eat a fibrous diet unlike pre-transplant when it was restricted to prevent overworking my failed kidney. I was to monitor myself for warning signs that my body was rejecting the kidney. This included pain, swelling, and flu-like symptoms.

The discharge nurse coordinator told me to relax and give myself adequate time to recover once home…. *"And God himself shall be with them, and be their God. And God shall wipe away all tears from their eyes; and there shall be no more death, neither sorrow, nor crying, neither shall there be any more pain: for the former things are passed away."*

Revelations 21: 3-4

I was expected to do lab work weekly for the first two months after the transplant so the team could continue to monitor my new kidney function. A church member who lived near me who was retired offered to take me to the lab facility near home. This was a Godsend. Living alone with a chronic health condition can be challenging. Having a support system is so important and over the years the support of good friends has been invaluable and something I treasure. With the risk of skin cancer, I was to see a dermatologist once a year to check my skin. I was also to check my skin periodically for any new spots, marks, moles or other changes.

I was cautioned not to have a large number of visitors during the first 6-8 weeks after surgery, and ask family members and friends who may have colds or infections to stay away. Being on a rigid schedule of immunosuppressants weakens the immune system, so the coordinator told me to pace myself, rest often and avoid crowded places including church, theaters and malls. I had to avoid eating from salad bars as they can harbor bacteria. To this day, friends still cannot understand why I refuse to eat from the open salad or food bars in restaurants, supermarkets or cafeterias. The high dose of prednisone I was on could contribute to weight gain so I kept a close watch on my weight and did my yoga workout every day. I could not take a shower for about 3-4 weeks until the drain was removed. That was a bummer. Who knew taking a shower was such a luxury. A home health nurse came twice a week to check the drain and dressing. She also changed the dressing as needed.

I contacted my professor and told her I was home and would start working on further revisions since I would now have more time while recuperating at home. She was happy I was home, but surprised I was going to resume working on the dissertation so quickly. I told her that I was resting for two weeks but had to take advantage of this time off as it gave me more time to focus with no distractions. She told me I was an amazing and strong woman.

October 26th arrived, three days after my discharge from the hospital and my birthday. My new kidney and just being home were the best birthday gifts ever! I had a new lease on life and I was in euphoria. I received quite a number of birthday cards and gift baskets. The staff from Johns Hopkins sent me a card signed by my transplant team and all the nurses who had taken care of me. It meant a lot. I spent a quiet day at home on my birthday and basked in the love of calls, cards and gift baskets from friends, my cousins, older brother and my aunt Hazel.

I was getting stronger each day and after input from both advisors, completed the final edits in early November. I had my follow-up visit with Dr. Geetha at the Bayview clinic rather than the transplant center since I was a vasculitis patient. I was still reasonably well since my transplant and as I relayed to her, I had noticed overall improvement in my energy level. My lab work showed my new kidney's function continued to improve. Dr. Geetha increased the dosage of one of my transplant medications as the level appeared low. My ureteral stent and peritoneal dialysis catheter was scheduled to be removed in two weeks. She noted my magnesium level was low so started me on magnesium supplementation. I still continue to take a magnesium supplement due to the loss as a result of the transplant medications.

Thanksgiving 2009 Post Transplant

Thanksgiving Day dawned. I decided to spend Thanksgiving quietly at home. It was only one month after my transplant, so I was still recuperating. Even though I was alone on Thanksgiving I had much to be thankful to God for that day and always. I cried at being alone, but wiped away the tears as I thought of the wonderful gift God had bestowed on me and the friends (angels) he had put in my path to see me through this challenging journey.

I decided to make the apple walnut pudding I had set out to make on the day I was called to receive my new kidney, oxtail stew, and watch movies. No school work that day. It was a day to celebrate! It was actually very dreary outside, but I heard from a lot of good friends, my cousins and felt good and warm inside.

December arrived and I continued to get stronger. Dr. Geetha continued to adjust my medications depending on my weekly labs. My prednisone levels were again lowered, for which I was thankful. The higher dosage contributed to weight gain. The dosage was still at a high level post-transplant and she explained it would be gradually reduced as I continued to do well. She noted that my umbilical hernia was no longer present. I was now scheduled to do lab work every two weeks versus every week. Christmas eve I spent almost all morning at Johns Hopkins on a follow-up appointment. I took a Christmas present for Dr. Geetha and Jamaican Christmas black cake for her and the staff. They were so delighted. It gave me great pleasure to show them how much I appreciated their support. Like Thanksgiving, I spent a quiet time at home that Christmas, exchanging holiday greetings with friends and thanking God for his wonderful blessing of a new kidney. While I was recovering those 3 months, I would arise each morning and rush to the landing of my home to watch the sunrise above the woods in the back. I was so thankful to awake each morning, thanking God for his gift of life, and seeing the sunrise each morning held a renewed meaning. Even now, when I awake, I go the landing to watch the sunrise and know that I can face the day, no matter what it may bring.

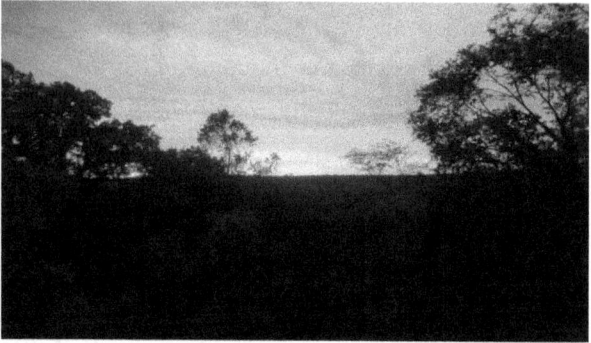

View of the Sunrise, December 2009

Happy New Year 2010

The New Year arrived and I felt full of hope. I received a special gift card from a former high school friend. It arrived just in time to help with expenses. God was indeed good in providing supportive friends. I returned to work on the third week in January, three months after my transplant surgery.

Snowmageddon in February 2010

It was not quite a month after my return to work that the North Eastern states including Washington D.C. and Maryland were hit by a big winter storm, February 5-6th. The 'Snowmageddon' storm as referred to by President Obama was the biggest snowstorm in nearly 90 years and was the 2nd, 3rd and even 4th significant winter storm for some parts of the Mid-Atlantic States that winter. It was predicted to snow, but no one knew we would get that much snow. In Maryland where I lived we received over 20 inches of snow. It covered the mailbox and the lower half of my car. Following my mother's example, during the winter season, my pantry was always stocked. The teenagers in my neighborhood made good pocket money that winter. I was so thankful to see them, as they came by to shovel me out. It took days for the neighborhoods to dig out. Many roads were closed and were impassable due to the heavy snow across Southern Pennsylvania and Maryland. It was quite a phenomenon.

With my new lease on life, on my return to work, I realized I no longer needed to endure the way things were going at my company. I no longer felt engaged. The culture was no longer appealing to me and I was getting more stressed. By the end of February, I had completed all my edits and my dissertation was accepted by my committee. With my final dissertation defense scheduled for March 2010, I was determined to make a change. I proactively began looking for other job opportunities more aligned with my career goals.

I began experiencing pain in my lower leg and lesions which my dermatologist had biopsied. My primary care doctor prescribed oxycodone to help control the pain at bedtime. I also started experiencing increased hair loss again. I could not determine if this was as a result of the stress at work or reaction from my medication. On my follow-up visit with Dr. Geetha near the end of January she lowered the dosage of my prednisone. Thankfully my weight was also lowering with the reduced dosages.

The biopsy of my lesions revealed they were benign. Dr. Geetha realized I was very sensitive to Prograf one of my transplant medications so she reduced the dosage. The lesions eventually disappeared. I have been on the lowered dosage ever since.

CHAPTER 7

GRADUATION—DR. BROWN

March arrived and I successfully defended my dissertation at Virginia Tech. It was all over in a couple of hours. I was not nervous, but rather enjoyed the dialogue with the committee members. It was surreal. After a couple of hours discussing my investigative findings on the "Consequences of Telecommuting: The Affects and Effects on Non-Telecommuters" I became Dr. Judith Brown!!!! Driving home that evening, I was so happy but my heart also ached. I had hoped my parents were alive to share the news with them.

My advisor sent me an email a few days later. She wanted me to enter my research into the 2010 26th annual Graduate Student Associate Research Symposium. I decided to enter the competition even though I was competing against primarily engineers at the Blacksburg campus. There were 205 oral presentations, posters, and videos presented at the symposium. A few weeks later I received an email that my research abstract was among the finalists chosen. On March 24th, I chose to do a video conference presentation of my research since I was located at the Northern Virginia location, quite a distance from the Blacksburg main campus. After my video conference, I returned to work. I was glad I was selected but I figured one of the engineering students would win. A couple days of days later I received a call from my advisor. She was very excited. I was awarded first place in the research symposium and received $500 and a certificate. I was over the moon. I could not wait to share the news with my Aunt and close friends.

My graduate ceremony was scheduled for May and I was at the school formatting my dissertation for publication when the head of the school, came up behind me and said she had a request. Would I consider representing the school as the student speaker at the ceremony? I just stared at her mouth agape. At this juncture I was so looking forward to completing the publishing of my dissertation, and just to walk across the stage and accept my degree. Student speaker?!…oh my. I told her I would think about it, but both her and my advisor said there was not much time as my entry had to be in by the end of that week. On my return to the office, I called and told her yes, I would be honored. I thought about what all my peers and I had been through to reach this milestone. I wanted to share this with others. I began drafting my speech and asked my advisor and Rafael to review. I only had

5 minutes to speak and wanted to ensure I covered the key highlights for the audience. After submission to the graduation committee, I awaited the verdict.

I did not have long to wait. A few days later, I received a call from the head of the graduation committee that I was one of the finalists and to come to the school to present my speech. I practiced my speech with my Aunt and Cam before I went before the committee. The day of the presentation I was pretty upbeat. During my presentation I saw the head of the committee wipe away tears. The next day I received another call. I was selected to deliver the Graduate Student Commencement Speech. I was so thrilled. I could not wait to share the wonderful news with my close friends and my doctors. I had my follow-up appointment at Johns Hopkins with Dr. Geetha in early April. I shared the good news with her on being chosen as the student speaker at my graduation and also receiving the research award. She was so delighted and gave me a big hug. My lab work also revealed I continued to do well with no episodes of rejection or renal vasculitis which was still in remission. I was to continue my triple immunosuppression medications program: Prograf, Mycophenolate and Prednisone to prevent rejection.

A few weeks later the Virginia Tech News carried a feature article on the upcoming graduate commencement in which I was featured.

Virginia Tech News, April 29, 2010
Community Spirit: Commencement

I have the honor of introducing the 2010 Student Speaker, Judith May Octavia Brown, who will receive her Ph.D. in Human Development at Commencement. Judith was born in Jamaica, and now resides in Washington, Maryland. She is a Senior Compliance Specialist for McNeil Technologies, where she has over fourteen years' experience as a researcher, analyst, and compliance specialist. Her work involves identifying the major challenges facing Human Resources professionals, managers, and employees in both the public and private sectors, and developing products and resources to enhance their individual and organizational performance. Judith earned a Master's Degree in Human Resource Management at the University of Maryland in 1995 and her Bachelor's Degree, magna cum laude, in History and Social Sciences from the University of the West Indies in 1987. She completed her dissertation while meeting the health challenges of unplanned kidney disease resulting in a successful kidney transplant in October 2009.

Graduation was scheduled for Sunday, May 16th. I took a few days off prior to graduation to de-stress, do a spa treatment and go over my speech. On the morning of graduation, I awoke excited and said a prayer of Thanksgiving. I called my aunt and she said she wished she could be there. I told her I would be thinking of her and my parents when giving my speech.

Close friends and former high school friends from Maryland, New York and Boston were going to be in attendance. I had invited my Mom's cousin and Dr. Osman. Dr. Geetha was unable to attend.

As we were assembling to go onstage, my advisor Claire asked if I was feeling nervous. I told her actually I did not. I felt so calm, which was unusual. When I was introduced to speak, I calmly walked to the podium:

Judith Brown

SUCCEEDING DESPITE TREMENDOUS OBSTACLES
By JUDITH M.O. BROWN
Valedictorian Speaker

President Steger and Vice President and Dean of Graduate Education DePauw, Trustees, Faculty, family, friends and fellow graduates, I am truly honored to speak to you on this momentous day of celebration.

First, I would like to thank the administration and faculty at the National Capital Region of Virginia Polytechnic Institute and State University for the hard work and dedication on our behalf. You have generously given your time and scholarship, and have supported me and my fellow graduates along a challenging and rewarding journey. We received the highest quality education here at Virginia Tech, while the understanding and encouragement you provided were essential to the ultimate achievement of our degrees, as we juggled multiple roles.

Second, a profound thanks to all of our family and friends who supported us throughout this journey, tolerated our crazy schedules, our excuses for not attending family or social functions, going to the movies, postponing vacations, and as one of my classmates said, "picked me up off the floor" as we stressed over deadlines.

Bruce Jenner, Olympic gold medalist said, "Realize that the reason most people fail isn't because of the competition but because of the limits they place upon themselves, allowing defeat to take over. Take responsibility for your destiny. You can come up with a performance, if you can reach down and dig deep enough into your competitive soul. You can overcome tremendous obstacles. "

Personally I can relate to this exhortation, having overcome a serious medical condition to be able to proudly stand before you today. At times I faltered, but would always hear my late mother's voice saying "Chin up, my girl." Mom and Dad, I did it. I refused to give up, and always told myself there is a light at the end of the tunnel. I know you, my fellow graduates, are also reflecting on the obstacles and challenges you had to overcome to be here today, refusing to place limitations on what you could achieve. You can now all say with me, "Wow! I made it."

> *Fellow graduates, today we have finished something, yet it is also the beginning of other journeys, of new dreams and opportunities. The charge of our University's motto is Ut Prosim (That I May Serve). Sometimes I think it is ironic that often in each endeavor of our academic lives we learn and grow and achieve the highest level possible in that institution and then we graduate...*
>
> *However, the opportunity exists for us to keep climbing; it is an endless ladder to heights we have never achieved before, to numerous paths opening in front of us! And if it is that way, I urge you to make sure that you are on a ladder you truly want to be, one that you have passion for; and never forget to be an inspiration, to motivate and help others as you continue to pursue your goals and dreams.*
>
> *Onward, my fellow graduates of 2010!*

The applause was deafening. After I received the degree and the ceremony ended, I was hugged by my fellow graduates and greeted with hugs and kisses from friends. Even though I had invited

Dr. Osman, I wasn't sure he would have been able to make it. I was pleasantly surprised when I heard his voice behind me. He gave me a hug and congratulated me. Without his early intervention and quick diagnosis I would not have been able to make that speech and walk across that stage. I forever will be grateful to him.

I went out to a celebration luncheon with my dear friends who attended the ceremony. I was so happy, and went to sleep that night thanking God for a perfect day and his perfect grace.

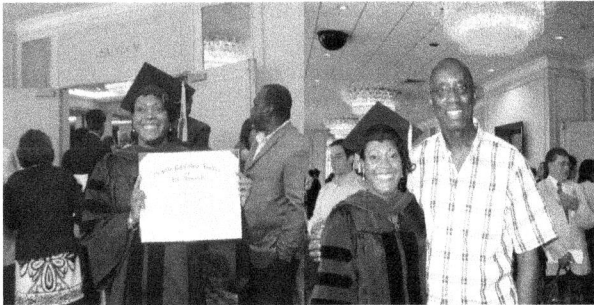

| Doctoral Degree at Graduation May 16, 2010 | With Dr. Osman at Graduation May 16, 2010 |

I continued to receive many gifts, including gift cards from friends and family after my graduation. I felt so loved and appreciated. At my work, they had a surprise luncheon for me and presented me with an iPod with Congrats Dr. Judith Brown engraved and ITunes gift cards. I had always wanted one and was so delighted.

In the coming months I continued working fulltime. My health remained reasonably well post-transplant. While I had spent the last four years experiencing devastating health challenges, and losing a boyfriend, I also viewed it as blessing for how it made me more appreciative of life. My surgeon had told me that even with the transplant, there was no guarantee my vasculitis would not return. Even though I was being asked by leadership to lead more formal training efforts at work, and things only got busier, I was not feeling fulfilled. I actively asked professional connections to let me know of suitable opportunities and kept up my search. I started my bucket list in 2007 after my diagnosis of renal vasculitis. Even though I had travelled to Europe prior to my diagnosis for work conferences and did some sightseeing, my bucket list really began with my trip to Ireland. I had felt I would wait to really travel to certain dream places only after I was in a serious relationship or married. I no longer felt that way after my diagnosis. I realized that every day was precious and I should not put off my passions or let my happiness depend on being in any relationship except with God.

CHAPTER 8

POST-TRANSPLANT, PHD - LIFE CHANGES

I had written articles as a requirement of my job as a Human Resources (HR) Professional, which were published in various HR Journals and HR Websites. In July of 2010, I was contacted by the editor of Digicast Productions in Australia to reprint an article I had written on *Employee Orientations: Keeping New Employees On Board* for HR Website, The Balance Careers. The editor of Digicast not only reprinted my article but also interviewed me on the subject of the importance of employee orientation in organizations. I felt more empowered to explore more of my life passions, which included writing, mentoring others and travelling. As a result of my writing not only for Digicast but later HR Matters, (now called Accelerate, the HR Magazine of Malaysia), I made more professional connections. I was being contacted by students working on projects to others who sought my advice on how to grow their careers. I saw now that my life could mean so much more.

I resumed my bucket list by planning what I called *My Celebration of Life*. On the advice of my cousin, I reached out to her travel agent Susan of AAA, who now has become my travel agent and friend. I had decided to go Hawaii. She helped me plan my trip, which was the "Best of Hawaii," exploring the four major islands: *Oahu, Kauai, Maui and the Big Island*. I scheduled my trip for two weeks after Christmas through after the New Year. I wanted to properly celebrate my gift of life and achievement of my PhD.

October 2010 Birthday Celebrations

For my birthday celebration I began what has become a tradition of celebrating the entire month. I had my kidney transplant the on the 10th so Dr. Geetha always refer to it as my Birthday Month. Each day I would do something special for myself, no matter how small. I had a massage and a facial starting the first day of October and weekly lunch dates with friends. On my actual Birthday on the 26th, I went in late to work as Rafael took me to lunch to celebrate. I gave God thanks for a blessed year.

Hawaii: Celebration of Life

A few days after Christmas, 2010, I departed for my trip to Hawaii. I spent two weeks island hopping from Oahu, to Kauai, Maui and the Big Island. It was indeed a wonderful celebration. I went canoeing on Kauai, enjoyed a luau event on Maui and even a helicopter ride over the volcanic Big Island. The scenery was absolutely beautiful, and I ate wonderful fresh seafood and fruit galore.

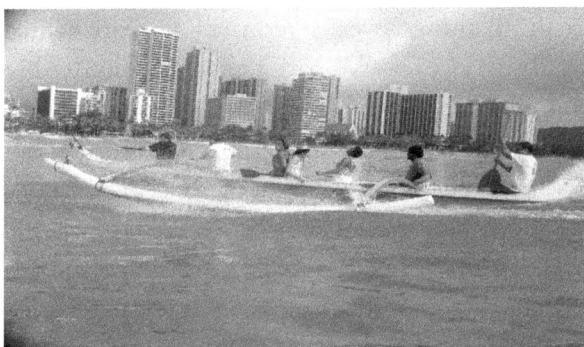

Canoeing at Kauai, 2011

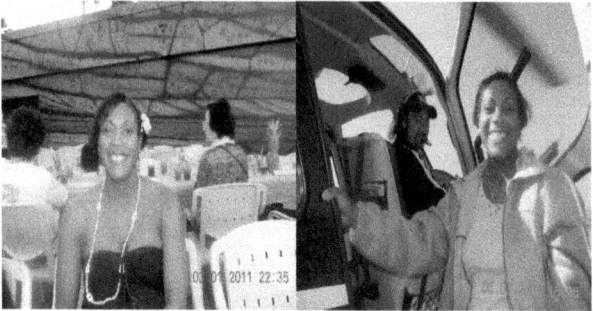

Luau on   Helicopter ride on Big
Maui , 2011   Island, 2011

After I came back from Hawaii I had a lot of time
to think things over. I returned to work which
was busy as ever. We had a change of leadership
and experienced a merger. I had been promised a
promotion with a leadership role in Training, but
as time went on, my boss kept making excuses.
By May, after getting nowhere after confronting
him, I realized I had to make a decision. I did not
like the direction the company was taking. My lab
work which I now had to do every month revealed
my creatine levels were again increasing. Dr.
Geetha became concerned and said she was going
to request I do a biopsy to see if I was experiencing a rejection. My blood pressure was high and
she ordered me to do a 24 hour urine test. I had
to carry a container to work to collect my urine so
she could evaluate my urine output over 24 hour
period. I told her I was experiencing some stress at
work and she repeated what she had told me the

first time we met after my diagnosis, "you have to strive to minimize the stress in your life" or your vasculitis may return. I decided to call my health insurance company to see what would be the cost of paying for COBRA if I should terminate my employment. I talked it over with Rafael, and told him the stress was getting too much for me and was beginning to affect my health. I told him I planned on resigning and look for something else, even if temporary until I figured out what direction to take regarding a better career opportunity. I decided to take a break for a couple months, and explore working part-time until something suitable came along. He said he would support me in my decision.

I remember I handed in my resignation after the Mother's Day weekend. I was fearful of making a change, but knew I could not stay much longer as the stress was affecting my health. A few of my peers thought I was making a mistake, but I told them the longer I stayed the worst it would become. I had met with a few recruiters who advised me to explore consultancy work to see if I would like it. I first decided to undergo a surgical procedure to address problems I was having with fibroids. I had the surgery in July and it went well. After recuperating at home, I resumed exploring job opportunities. Rafael would pass on any leads he came across. Whenever I felt despondent at not finding anything suitable, he would tell me, "Giving up is not an option."

Early in the New Year of 2012, he sent me an email with a quote which gave me further motivation not to give up:

> *Each morning when I open my eyes I say to myself: I, not events, have the power to make me happy or unhappy today. I can choose which it shall be. Yesterday is dead, tomorrow hasn't arrived yet. I have just one day, today, and I'm going to be happy in it.*

~ Groucho Marx

I finally received a two year contract offer as Principal Consultant for a consultancy firm in mid – October in their Federal Systems Division. God never fails.

My health continued to improve and for the next two years I gained experience working as a consultant. As the two years winded down, I decided to look for a full-time position. This time I decided to search for a full-time position as I wanted the security of health coverage and leave the uncertainty of contract life. I received an offer from Lockheed Martin. Simultaneously, I was also offered a position with the CIA. After seeking God's guidance, I accepted the offer at Lockheed

Martin which offered great benefits. The research position intrigued me and it was an area I always loved. I was back in the corporate world and began work at my new position in mid – September of 2013. I found my work at Lockheed quite fulfilling and impactful. I also had the opportunity to work from home at least two days a week. I kept busy with work and sometimes it got overwhelming, but being a "Type A" personality I know I am at fault for not taking more down time.

Early November, I started feeling unwell. I thought I was coming down with the flu. I did my monthly labs that Saturday. Even though I was feeling unwell, I went to work. I had just started the new position and did not want to be missing work so soon. I was in a staff meeting on Monday and felt worse. I went to the medical center and the nurse checked my blood pressure which was high. She told me to rest and she would take my pressure again. When I returned to my desk, Dr. Geetha called. She was concerned. She had received my labs and my creatine levels had increased, and my white cell count was over 23,000. I told her I was not feeling well. She said she was going to call Dr. Osman to coordinate me going to the hospital. Dr. Osman called me back and instructed me to go straight to the emergency room at Southern Maryland hospital so I would get immediate attention. He had called ahead to the hospital. My boss offered to drive me but I told her I would be okay to drive. I did not want to leave my car in the garage at work. I told her I would call when I arrived at the hospital.

On my arrival, I was admitted after they started me on intravenous antibiotics in the emergency room. I called my girlfriend Jean as Rafael was not in town. Jean came right after dropping off her kids at home after picking them up from school. After running tests, they discovered I actually had a urinary tract infection. With my transplanted kidney close to my urinary tract, this was potentially dangerous. I remained in the hospital for a week on intravenous antibiotics. I reached out to my Sister-in-law to let her know what happened. She sent my younger brother with toiletries, as I had driven to the hospital straight from work. I was finally released to go home when my creatine numbers and white cell count began to fall. I was switched to oral antibiotics when I was discharged. I remained at home for a week resting, then returned to work. That was a close call. My creatine numbers never went back to the levels they were before the infection. Dr. Geetha explained that after an infection the creatine levels sometimes do not return to their previous levels. The important thing was to aim to prevent another infection. I have been vigilant ever since to avoid infections as much as I am able.

CHAPTER 9

TURNING 50

In October 2014, I was turning 50. I wanted to celebrate this milestone in a special way. I decided to add Australia to my bucket list. I always wanted to travel there and meet a Koala bear face to face. They were so adorable. I reached out to Susan my travel agent and began making plans for my trip. October arrived and I was off. I had an awesome time, one of my best birthday trips. Susan had shared my birthday with the tour guide, so it was a pleasant surprise that at each of the resorts during my birthday week, the hotel staff left chocolate and in one case two bottles of champagne when we arrived in Cairns. Considering I do not drink, I shared this with members of my tour group. On the chartered flight from Melbourne to Sidney the pilot and crew sang "Happy Birthday" to me and the flight attendant presented me with a chocolate cupcake with a birthday candle. I even got to hug a Koala bear on my birthday – Yay!!! My dream had come true (Australia is one day ahead of the U.S.A) so even though it was the 27th in Australia, it was actually the 26th in the U.S.A. The morning after my birthday I took a ride in a hot air balloon. That was an experience. I got to see the sunrise while riding in a hot air balloon. It was an absolutely grand birthday trip!

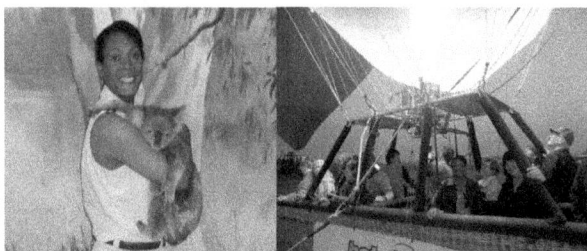

Hugging a Koala Bear - October 27, 2014

Riding in a Hot Air Balloon - October 28, 2014

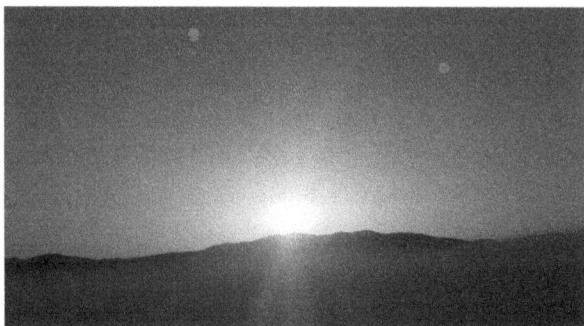

Sunrise watch from Hot Air Balloon – Australia, October 28, 2014

2015 dawned. The year started out uneventful, but that all changed in February. The Washington DC area experienced another whopping winter storm. The biggest since the snowmaggedon in 2010. Despite a very slow start, the winter of 2014-2015 was the longest I remembered. From mid-February through the first half of March 2015, winter took hold and would not let go. The Church leadership cancelled services at my congregation due to the inclement weather. Imagine winter in spring! Ice melt and salt was in short supply. I was able to get some from a local store owner who shared some of his personal supply with me. When Rafael called to check on me and I told him I only had a small supply, he came and brought one of his own bags from home. He had the foresight and bought some extra bags a few days before the rush on ice melt and salt. Even the road crews that usually placed ice salt on the streets were running out of supply. It was not just snowing, but also was very icy. He put some ice melt down on the front steps and on the driveway. I was so thankful to see him.

After the dramatic winter in 2015, my thoughts turned to the upcoming 67th Annual Society for Human Resources Management (SHRM) Conference. It was being held in Las Vegas. I found the topics on the program planned for 2015 on diversity and workforce planning of interest. I also planned on having dinner with Rita, a close friend and former worker who lived in Nevada. I had not seen her in years, and was looking forward to seeing her. SHRM also was sponsoring a live concert with Jennifer Hudson, one of my favorite singers. I was so excited.

The conference was one of the best I ever attended: It was packed with informative sessions and dynamic speakers such as Mika Brzezinski of MSNBC and Mike 'Coach K' Krzyzewski iconic Duke University basketball coach. Hanging out with Rita and attending the Jennifer Hudson concert was the icing on the cake! Jennifer Hudson's performance was awesome. Everyone was on their feet, including moi, singing and dancing to every song. But that was not the end. While sitting in my last session, I heard an announcement for me to come to the auditorium where all the vendors were located. I then got a text saying I had won a TV. I thought it was a hoax at first. The session was almost over so I went over to the auditorium to investigate. Going along with the Vegas theme, all the vendors at the conference offered all attendees the opportunity to enter drawings for their products. I never usually won anything of significance so I had put the idea of winning anything out of my mind. When I arrived at the auditorium, vendors were packing up and I ran to the vendor who had the TV drawing. The lady who was there verified my identity and said I had won the LG LED TV! I just jumped up and down and hugged her. She said it would be shipped to me via Federal Express. I texted Rafael and he could not believe it. I do not gamble and he could not believe I won this 52 inch LED TV so easily. On my flight back to Maryland after the conference was over, I was over the moon reliving my experiences at the conference. The true icing on the cake was winning that LED TV.

October 10th arrived and also my 5 year anniversary since my kidney transplant. I was experiencing good health and gave God thanks for watching over me and keeping hold of me. On my birthday on the 26th I received many well wishes from friends and family. I was feeling so blessed. In December, based on the encouragement of friends, I made a decision to write my memoirs on my journey. I decided to write about living with vasculitis, with all the challenges and triumphs I experience. They kept telling me over the years my story was an inspiration to others. I decided to take the plunge, but would not focus on my writing until the fall of 2018.

In early 2016, my boss at Lockheed hinted there were major changes that were going to take place. Layoffs began to occur. Writing my memoirs was placed on the back burner. My former colleague who had relocated to Colorado and an excellent research analyst was one of those laid off. Things were becoming very scary. My boss shared with me that she suspected our research group was in jeopardy hence why she decided to take early retirement. She encouraged me to start looking for another position. My heart was heavy. I had been there three years. I thought Lockheed would be my last career stop. I had not planned on looking for another opportunity at this stage of my life and wondered what God's plan was. I spoke to Rafael about the situation. He shared with me that he thought I should consider working with the Federal Government as there would be better security. I would be assured of continued health care unlike in the private sector. I considered this and realized he was correct. With my chronic health condition, I had to be strategic in my next job search. I had to face reality. My boss also agreed when I began my search. Her husband worked for the Federal Government and she confirmed what Rafael said. She offered to be a reference as I conducted my search for federal positions.

On my way in to work one morning in May, I received a call from the Navy regarding my application. I went in for an interview and went home thinking this was a great opportunity to get my foot in the door and to have a career in the Federal Government. I prayed to God asking for His guidance in making the right decision. A few days after the interview, I received a call from the staffing specialist with an offer for the position as an HR Specialist. I was so happy to share the news with

Rafael who was also thrilled. He advised me on negotiating an acceptable salary and they accepted my offer. I eventually on boarded as a civilian with the Navy in July 2016. I had made plans with my travel agent to go to Cuba prior to accepting the position at the Navy. It was another adventure I wanted to add to my bucket list. I thought it would be another great birthday gift to me.

My travel agent had made the arrangements for me to go on a small group tour. I had to get permission from the Navy to make the trip to Cuba. Only People to People tours were acceptable and my small group tour fell into that category. I was granted permission.

A couple weeks before my trip I did my monthly lab work. I chose to do it at the Quest Diagnostics near work rather than the one nearest home where I always did my lab work. I thought it would be more convenient. A couple of days later, Dr. Geetha called. My creatine level had suddenly risen rather high. She wanted me to do a biopsy. I told her no. I felt fine. This was not possible. I was leaving for Cuba in another week. I told her I wanted to retake the lab work. It must be a fluke. I called Dr. Osman's office and asked him to talk to her. I did not feel a biopsy was necessary. I was not missing my trip. This was not happening. He asked me about the lab work. I told him I had taken it at the Quest near my office. He said he would have another lab request faxed to my regular center near home. I was to go there and redo the test. He said sometimes doing lab work at different centers can generate different results, so he wanted me to go back to my regular center. I went to my usual center the Friday morning. I was scheduled to depart for Cuba the next day. He had ordered it STAT for urgency. I was determined to go to Cuba, so I did not call Susan my travel agent to alert her to reschedule. Aware of my health challenges, she always had me take out travel insurance whenever I went on my trips in the event there was a medical emergency. I felt fine. I somehow knew the lab work would reveal normal levels.

I was getting dressed for my departure to the airport when Dr. Geetha called. I can always tell by the tone of her voice if something was wrong, and her tone was upbeat. I let out a sigh of relief. My creatine level had actually dropped to 1.2, which was even below my usual baseline range of 1.7!!! I was ecstatic and laughed. I told Dr. Geetha I was getting dressed to depart to the airport. She wished me a wonderful and safe trip. I thanked God for his intervention. I was on my way to Cuba.

My 8 day stay in Cuba is an experience I will never forget. The rich culture, meeting the local artists in their studios, and the colonial architecture. Even though I stayed in a lovely 5 star hotel in Havana, I particularly liked my stay in a casa particular, a privately owned bed and breakfast run by a Cuban family in the city of Cienfuegos. It offered a more personal experience. The meals at paladares, family owned restaurants that served local Cuban cuisine, were also quite delicious. Upon learnng that I loved plantains, my tour companions would laugh and always passed me the plate of plantains first wherever it was served as an appetizer.

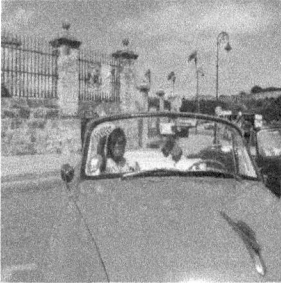

Cuban vintage car   Sunrise view over
                              Cienfuegos

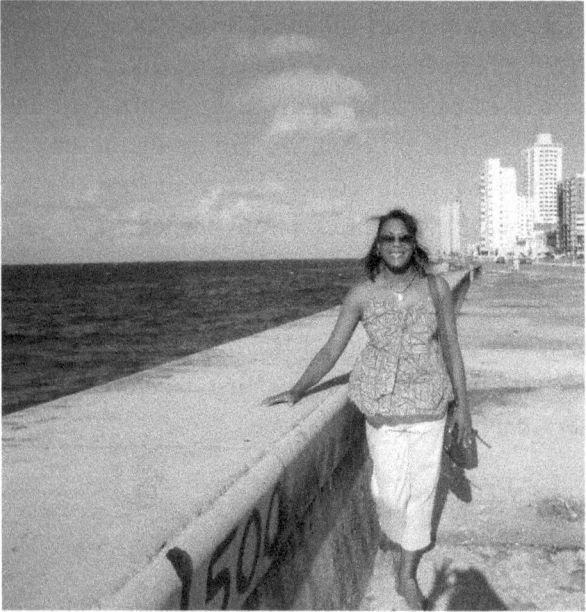

Along the Malecon, Havana, Cuba

By early May 2017, I was with the Navy for eight months. Work was going well. I worked a compressed work schedule, which meant I had every other Friday off. This flexibility allowed me to schedule my 4 month appointments with Dr. Osman and some of my other doctors on the Fridays I was off. This was extremely helpful so I would not need to use up sick leave for my frequent doctor visits. I decided to revisit the writing of my memoirs.

My vasculitis and kidney condition had been the major health challenges I had to face up to this point. I had a procedure done in 2011 to shrink my fibroids which had proved to be very successful. I had not had any problems since then. Alas, this was the calm before the storm.

I found myself experiencing persistent bleeding which continued past two weeks. I became alarmed as I thought after I turned 50 my cycle would slow down. I started to double-up on my iron tablets and called my gynecologist's office. She was not in the office so I left an urgent message with the nurse to let her know what was happening. She returned my call later that day. She explained that in some women the bleeding accelerated then eventually slowed down. As a precaution she had me come in for an examination.

At the visit she gave me a referral to schedule an ultrasound. The bleeding had lessened, but with my history of fibroids she wanted to eliminate any resurgence as a reason for the bleeding. She said to continue taking the iron twice a day to prevent anemia. I went to an appointment the following morning and work afterwards. I anxiously awaited the results of the ultrasound.

A few days later my gynecologist called. The ultrasound showed a new growth. She indicated she wanted to schedule the removal of the fibroid and had me make an appointment with the surgical nurse. I could not believe I was going through this again. I thought those days were in the past.

The embolization procedure I did in 2011 was supposed to take care of my fibroids. Although it was not a 100 percent guarantee, I had an uneventful six years so I felt I was safe. I figured after I turned 50, I would go into menopause with no more issues. This was the last thing I expected.

I prayed this procedure would be the final hurdle before things finally slowed down. I made the appointment with the surgical nurse for May 12th a few days before Mother's Day. The outpatient procedure was scheduled to take place at Southern Maryland Hospital. I would not be required to stay overnight. Sister Johnson, a close friend at church offered to accompany me as I was to be under general anesthesia.

The procedure went well. It only took a couple of hours. I awoke in the recovery room with some moderate pain. I was on IV and the nurses would periodically come by to check my vitals. They wanted to ensure I was stable before being discharged. Sister Johnson helped me dress after picking up my pain medication from the pharmacy. I was to return for a post-operation follow-up with my gynecologist in another week. I was anxious to get the details from her about the entire procedure. I actually expected to be in more pain as she was supposed to have also conducted a procedure, endometrial ablation to remove my uterus lining which would prevent any future bleeding.

I remained at home a week after the procedure to rest and recuperate. I followed up with her the following week. The visit was unexpected to say the least. She started out by saying that the fibroid she removed was benign but she had not conducted the endometrial ablation as there was something unusual about the lining of my uterus. It had a yellowish color. The pathologist also did not know what was wrong as "he had not seen this before." He determined it was not malignant but could not provide a definitive diagnosis. She also told me she had not seen this before in a uterus lining but was recommending I do a hysterectomy in the event it did become malignant later on. I balked at this idea. If she had no idea what was wrong with my uterus lining, I was not going to do a hysterectomy, a drastic procedure without having a definite answer. I told her I would think about it, but at that moment made up my mind to get another opinion.

I spoke to both Francesca and Rafael who agreed with me. I called the office of the physician at Georgetown who had performed the embolization procedure in 2011. I explained the situation to the nurse and she said they would want me to do a repeat MRI and they would obtain the pathology report from my gynecologist. The earliest appointment I could get was in late June. I did the ultrasound in early June. I called and told my gynecologist I was going to get a second opinion. She agreed it was a good idea when I told her I was concerned with the pathology report's inconclusiveness.

During the wait time for my appointment in June at Georgetown, I conducted further research based on the pathology findings. I found nothing except it could be atypical and potentially lead to malignancy. I found comfort in knowing I was getting another opinion. The unknown was scary.

My appointment day finally arrived. When I arrived, I learned the physician had an unexpected family emergency, so I saw the attending physician. She examined the new MRI and pathology report. She was under the impression that it could be as a result of my vasculitis condition but could not offer anything conclusive. She suggested she would have the other physician I was to see originally look at the results upon his return. She promised he would call me with his diagnosis to prevent me driving back all the way down to Georgetown. I was disappointed he was not available but relieved he would still review the new MRI and pathology report on his return.

A few days passed and I received a call at home. It was the physician from Georgetown. He had reviewed the pathology report and MRI. He was glad the finding was not malignant He had actually spoken to the pathologist to get further clarification and because of my vasculitis history and weakened immune condition, he felt it was in my best interest to have the hysterectomy. He said that unlike other women, if I developed cancer it would be more aggressive and it would be harder to treat. My lower immune system would make it more difficult to fight cancer. I expressed my concern that I was in a new position at work and it was going to be a busy period in a few months. Recovery from a hysterectomy was estimated to take 6-8 weeks! How soon did he think I needed to do surgery? He said, "as soon as possible, but would not recommend putting it off past spring of the following year." I told him I would do the procedure in the spring of 2018.

I had a follow-up appointment with Dr. Osman that summer of 2017. My labs continued to show stable results. Thank goodness for that. Drama seemed to follow me. He asked how I was I feeling and I relayed the latest on my gynecological issues. He said based on the location of my new kidney it would be best I did the procedure at a larger hospital, preferably at Johns Hopkins where my transplant records were located and where the transplant team would be available during the proceedings. When I called my gynecologist, I expressed this concern and she agreed. She was only assigned to Southern Maryland, the local hospital. She recommended I see a specialist at the oncology gynecology center at Washington Hospital Center to discuss it further. She said she would contact them with the referral.

I made the appointment with the doctor at the oncology gynecology department. He had both the pathology results and the last MRI from June. He echoed what the physician at Georgetown said about doing the hysterectomy. He however noted that as I was at high risk due to my kidney transplant, he would recommend a robotic hysterectomy procedure. This was not as invasive and would only require small incisions. The recovery time would also be less than if I had to receive a larger incision. I was comforted by his detailed explanation and kindness. He recommended his former partner Dr. Davis who now worked at Johns Hopkins and was experienced in doing the robotic procedure. This procedure was not done at the Washington Hospital Center. He gave me her contact information and said he would also give her a call.

I left the appointment more hopeful. On my way home, I called the Johns Hopkins Oncology Gynecology Department to make an appointment to see Dr. Davis. I was able to get an appointment in January of 2008. My appointment day arrived. Initially on meeting Dr. Davis I felt at ease. However, she appeared so young, like a teenager. I was a little skeptical, even though I had done my investigation and she had great reviews on her experience and expertise. She was also quite personable. I went over my history with her and she confirmed she had spoken to the doctor at Washington Hospital Center. She examined me and explained the robotic surgical procedure if I chose to do the procedure. I told her I was still weary of doing something as drastic as a hysterectomy. Since my last MRI was in June, she requested I do a repeat MRI so she would have a recent image for examination. I did a repeat MRI and waited. A few days later, on my way home from work one evening, my phone rang and it was Dr. Davis. She had the results. The image showed a thickening in the area of my uterus which was not on the earlier image taken in June. She said this was not unusual in premenopausal women but with my medical history and the likelihood of the atypical findings becoming malignant, she also recommended doing a hysterectomy soon. I was alarmed at this prospect, as a hysterectomy was such a drastic measure. She said I could wait and do another MRI every few months to see if things changed. I told her I would think more about it and let her know my decision that week.

I decided to call my older brother who is in the medical field and discussed it with him. He also said that the risk of doing nothing was more than my fear of going into early menopause with doing the hysterectomy. He agreed with my doctors that with my weakened immune system if it became malignant, it would be more difficult for my body to fight off. I also spoke to my cousin Donna in Canada. She said her stepsister had this procedure and it was successful. I thought more about it. I was past childbearing age and the thought that if I did nothing and did develop uterine cancer, it would be too late to effectively treat, drove me to make the decision. I called Dr. Davis's office and told the surgical nurse I wanted to proceed with the surgery. The surgery was scheduled for February 27, 2018.

I started making the necessary preparations for the surgery. I spoke to my boss and let her know the time frame I would be out of office so she could prepare the team for my absence. I submitted the necessary paperwork for leave under the Family Medical Leave Act (FMLA). My co-workers were supportive. I also had to go for pre surgery testing. Some tests I did at my local lab near home and some at Johns Hopkins. As each day went by, with my research into the procedure and talks with my cousin, I was feeling less troubled and focused on the positives. I think my greatest fear was the thought of the loss of what I perceived as the center of my womanhood. I still wondered how I would feel and kept reading blog posts from women who had a hysterectomy with the robotic procedure. The majority were positive. That gave me some comfort. I decided to stock up on supplies and groceries that were nonperishable. I knew that I would not be able to drive for at least a month after the surgery. I also did a thorough cleaning of the house. I had friends who could help out in any emergency but I needed to prepare as much as I could so I would only need to reach out to them if necessary.

The weekend before the surgery I did my regular transplant lab work. My surgery pretest which I had completed the week prior was all okay and I had the green light for surgery. I was feeling a dull ache in my lower abdomen and thought it was my menstrual cycle coming. I never thought anything of it. My girlfriend Francesca had volunteered to accompany me to surgery and scheduled to take off the week following my surgery to stay at home with me. I was ever so happy and grateful for her kindness and friendship. The night before the surgery, I had just completed my bath which included my surgery preparation when my phone rang. I was going to ignore the call as no one I know usually calls me that late at night –it was ten o'clock. The caller id also showed "private number" which did not register until it clicked in my brain that it was Dr. Geetha. She was the only person who called that had a private number. I quickly answered. She quickly said Judith, how are you? I have your lab work and it is showing your creatine is running over 2.00 and your white cell count is very high. I said that is not possible. I just did my pre-surgery tests the week before and everything was normal. She kept pressing me if I felt okay. I said I did notice I had this dull ache in my lower abdomen which now had moved to my lower right side. It so happened that was the same side my transplanted kidney was located. I had not even thought of that. She said she had notified the surgeon as she did not think I should proceed with the surgery until we found out what was happening. At the same time my cell phone started to ring. I told Dr. Geetha to hold on. On answering my cell, I discovered it was Dr. Davis. I told Dr. Geetha who was on the other line and she said okay, glad Dr. Davis had gotten her message.

Dr. Davis proceeded to tell me she had received the message from Dr. Geetha. She said she was reluctant to postpone the surgery but based on the results of the new tests, she would need to, until we figured out what had suddenly changed to send my numbers off the charts. She wanted me to still come in as scheduled the next morning so they could examine me. I was to go to the transplant center. I called Francesca and told her what happened. She said she would come for me as previously arranged the next morning. I gave her the address they had given me, as Johns

Hopkins Hospital had varied address locations for the different centers. Fortunately, Francesca also works at Johns Hopkins, so it was easier for her to navigate.

I went to bed that night quite anxious. I did not sleep very well. What could have gone wrong in such a short time? The next morning Francesca came early. Since the surgery was postponed, I think I had a slice of toast and some tea before we departed. When we finally arrived at the admission area of the transplant center, they were expecting me. I was admitted. The transplant team began to run tests. My white blood cell count was elevated and I was running a fever. I was hooked up to an IV. My levels were still high and were continuing to climb. All tests came back negative. By this time the pain in my lower left abdomen was a continuous ache. The doctors were giving me antibiotics intravenously, but my levels would not go down. My white blood cell count continued to increase. Different team members kept coming and asking me questions. The left side of my abdomen hurt to the touch. They scheduled a kidney biopsy. The results came back negative for rejection. Eventually one of the senior transplant doctors surmised that the problem was not with my kidney transplant. He thought it best to consult with the gynecology oncology (Gyn Onco) team. The Gyn Onco team wanted to do an ultrasound of my lower abdomen.

By this time, I had been in the hospital a couple of days.

Francesca who lived nearby had gone home. I told her I would call to keep her posted. She was visiting when I was scheduled to do the ultrasound and accompanied me to the lab. We tried to make light of the moment. I said to Francesca that her friend was a medical phenomenon. Nothing that happened to me was ever regular or simple. She laughed. While in the lab I was prepped for the ultrasound. The technician started the test. After a few minutes she stopped and told me to remain still. She had gone to get the laboratory doctor to further examine the image. The doctor started operating the ultrasound and commented "you have a very active uterus." I was astonished. What is it? Francesca laughed, jokingly saying I must have a baby in there with three heads. The doctor finally said it looked as if I had an ovarian abscess on my right ovary. She would finalize the test and send the results to Dr. Davis.

After I was returned to my room, the Gyn Onco team along with Dr. Davis came to see me. She had the results. She commented that this was new to her. She had never come across a case like mine. She was going to schedule a laparoscopy to remove the abscess from my right ovary. The procedure was scheduled for the next day. At least I now knew what was causing this entire problem.

I asked Dr. Davis if I would still be scheduled for the hysterectomy, the procedure I had originally scheduled. She said we would revisit after I had recovered from this procedure.

The next day they came to take me down to surgery. During the surgery, Dr. Davis called in the transplant team to assist as the area around the right ovary was too close to the vessels attached to my transplanted organ. With their assistance, Dr. Davis was able to successfully navigate around the transplanted kidney to remove my right ovary with the abscess. After I awoke in the recovery room, one of the nurses came over and gave me pain medication when I indicated I was in pain. I was then taken back to my room. The doctors noticed that my inflammation and fever improved. I was switched to oral antibiotics which I tolerated well. They reduced the dosage of Mycophenolate, one of my transplant medications, to allow me to fight the inflammation more successfully. My kidney function and therefore my creatine levels also improved after I was given extra fluids intravenously.

I was eventually discharged on March 10th. I had been in the hospital for almost two weeks. I was instructed to stay hydrated with at least 64 ounces of water daily. This had become part of my daily routine since my transplant in 2009. Staying hydrated is important for my kidneys to remain healthy. I was to continue taking the oxycodone as needed for pain and the oral antibiotics for two more weeks then follow up with Dr. Davis in a week.

I was at home recuperating for a few days and taking the oxycodone as needed for pain. I noticed I felt extremely tired and I was out of breath just going to the restroom to wash-up. I slept almost all day and still woke up tired. I went to do my lab work during the time I was recuperating. A few days later Dr. Geetha called. It was again late at night. She was concerned. My sodium level had fallen below normal levels. I told her I was feeling very weak. She wanted me to go to the emergency room at Johns Hopkins as it would be best I returned to the transplant unit for evaluation. I reminded her that I lived an hour away and I was not sure who I could call at this late hour to take me. I decided to call Francesca. She lived an hour away but I had no one else I could call. I had friends who lived closer to me but I did not want to trouble them. I felt better calling Francesca. She did not hesitate. She had not yet gone to bed. I told her I was willing to wait until she got to my home. Due to the late hour, it took her less than an hour to arrive at my home since there was no traffic. When she arrived she assisted me to the car. We took off for downtown Baltimore. I kept thanking her over and over. She was my guardian angel. We got to the emergency room and I was immediately taken to a room. I told the nurse that my sodium level was low. The attending emergency room team attached an IV solution to aid in gradually correcting my sodium levels. Francesca would not leave my side. She sat in a chair beside my bed the entire night. How can one repay such a friend? A technician came and took blood work. Later the attending emergency room doctor came by. My white cell count was again elevated. Upon examination, they discovered that there was still some right pelvic fluid that collected as a result of the surgery. This was not abnormal post-operation. Early in the morning, I was transferred to the intensive care unit for further observation. Francesca then told me she had to go off to work. I felt so guilty. She had spent all night in the chair with little to no sleep. I knew she was exhausted. She said she had to attend an important meeting and had to go in.

While I was in intensive care all persons: nurses, doctors, attendants coming in and out had to wear masks and hazmat type cover-ups to prevent any germs entering the room. I was again on intravenous antibiotics. The transplant doctors were again in attendance. They were monitoring my vitals and having my blood drawn every 4 hours to check how well my sodium level was rising. The senior specialist explained that they had to raise the level gradually as they did not want to shock my system. I could not believe I was back in the hospital. I prayed for strength. Francesca called around lunch time and said she was on her way home. She had found it difficult to stay awake and after explaining to her boss that she had spent all night in the emergency room with a friend, her boss ordered her to go home. I was glad she was going home. I told her not to worry about me. I would call her if anything changed and the hospital had her number.

I was transferred from intensive care after my sodium levels stabilized back to the transplant unit. The nurses who came by joked if I missed them. I had only been discharged a week before! They monitored me to ensure my white cell count continued to decrease and that my sodium level remained at the baseline. The senior attending transplant doctor did not want to take another chance to send me home until he was sure I was 100 percent stable. I was finally discharged on March 19th. I had been in the hospital a week on this second admission. I was scheduled to follow-up with Dr. Davis the end of March.

On my follow-up visit with Dr. Davis, she checked the site of my laparoscopy surgery and said it was healing nicely. We discussed the rescheduling of my robotic hysterectomy. She wanted to wait at least six weeks so I could heal from this first procedure. I scheduled the surgery with the scheduling assistant for April 24th. I contacted my boss to let her know the new date. I had been out of the office now for two months. If I had to be honest, I did not miss it. I needed the break. I liked being home. I actually look forward to retirement when I can spend the days pursuing my passions: writing, catching up on reading, tending to my garden, volunteering, and travelling.

I remained at home recuperating for another month before it was back to Johns Hopkins and finally my robotic surgery originally scheduled two months prior. The whole experience was surreal.

The morning of the 24th dawned and Francesca came to get me. There were no phone calls the previous night with medical alarms. My last lab work indicated all was stable. We arrived at admission and I went through pre-operation procedures. Dr Davis came by to go over the surgical procedure with me one last time. Mentally I was now more prepared. I had more time to do my research and consider the benefits. The fears had subsided. God somehow had convinced me I was making the right decision after my ovarian dramatic episode. I would still have my left ovary intact with the hysterectomy which would help lessen the impact of onset menopause post hysterectomy. Studies reveal that ovaries continue to make small amounts of estrogen for years after menopause.

The surgery took approximately four hours and went smoothly. I stayed overnight and again Francesca stayed with me. In this case, there was another bed in the room so she could sleep more comfortably. I was discharged the next day after they determined all my vitals were stable and I could move around. I was taught to use a brace around my abdomen to help with the healing and to provide support for my movements.

Francesca took me home and spent a week to assist me. Her stay that week was most welcome. Having had two surgeries in such a short space of time took its toll on me. The pain was great at times. Francesca fixed my meals and would not allow me to go down the stairs. I restricted my movements to the adjoining bathroom and the landing. It was at my postop follow-up with Dr. Davis that she elaborated that there was a lot of scarring around my stomach lining after the previous surgery. She had to scrape away the scarring when performing the robotic hysterectomy, hence why I was experiencing more pain than was usual after this procedure. I was scheduled to return to work after the July 4th break, on July 9th. I recuperated at home for approximately eight weeks where I continued to heal.

I returned to work in July. Thankfully I remained in good health the rest of the year. I took care to rest as much as I could. That October was nine years since my transplant and I was rejoicing at God's continued blessing and watch over me. I applied and got accepted in a special leadership program at work which would open up more opportunities for my career.

I wanted to celebrate my ten year transplant anniversary in 2019 in a special way so I contacted Susan my travel agent for ideas. After going back and forth, she asked me what I thought of visiting Greece in the summer. It had wonderful reviews and was also listed as one of the best places to visit. On reviewing the tour itinerary, I was sold. The thought of the beaches of Mikonos, swimming in the Aegean Sea, Greek food and seeing the ancient historical sites was heavenly. I told her to proceed with the planning.

In the fall of 2018, Peg and I went on our annual road trip to the Apple House in Linden, Virginia. I bought a sign in the gift shop titled *"This is my Happy Place."* I placed it in my garden in the spring of 2019, which I consider my sanctuary. I had a challenging 2018 with my health so I prayed for a less dramatic 2019 as it related to my health. The 2019 New Year had a busy start at work. I renewed my focus on writing my memoirs. I also began attending the forums for my leadership program in February and looked forward to what would unfold for the rest of the year.

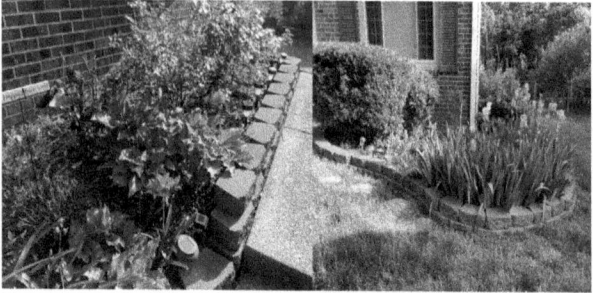

Judith's Spring Garden 2019

I continued to remain in good health for the remainder of 2019. God had been watching over me, and I am thankful for his grace and mercy. Summer arrived and I happily began packing for my two week trip to Greece near the end of June.

I arrived in Athens on June 27th and for the next 11 days I had a grand time. It was great visiting Athens, the country's capital where the Acropolis an ancient citadel dating back to the 5th century BC, sits high above the city. It was not an easy walk up the famed hill, but I made it and the reward was the 360-degree view of the city and the Aegean Sea beyond. I visited such ancient treasures as the Parthenon, one of Greece's more than 100 archaeological sites. I also ferried over to the beautiful island of Mykonos, relaxed on one of the stunning beaches and swam in the Aegean Sea. I also visited the volcanic island of Santorini. I love Mediterranean cuisine so I was in heaven eating authentic Gyros, eating classic Greek dishes such as moussaka and Greek salads.

On my final night on Santorini, I went on a sailboat cruise where I enjoyed a day of sailing, eating authentic cuisine, listening to Greek music and learning Greek dancing from a member of my tour group. The finale was watching the gorgeous fiery sunset. It was delightful marking my ten year transplant anniversary year visiting such a naturally beautiful and culturally rich country.

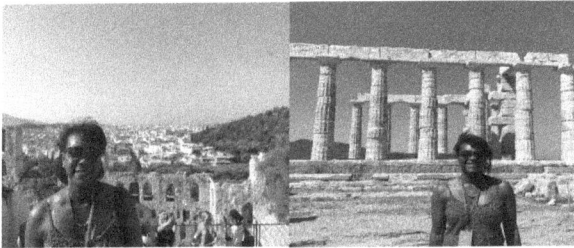

Visiting the Acropolis, Athens, June 2019

Visiting the Acropolis, Athens, June 2019

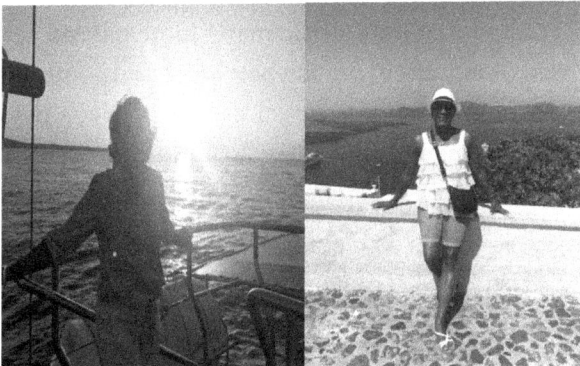

Sunset sail - Santorini, Greece, July 2019

Santorini, Greece, July 2019

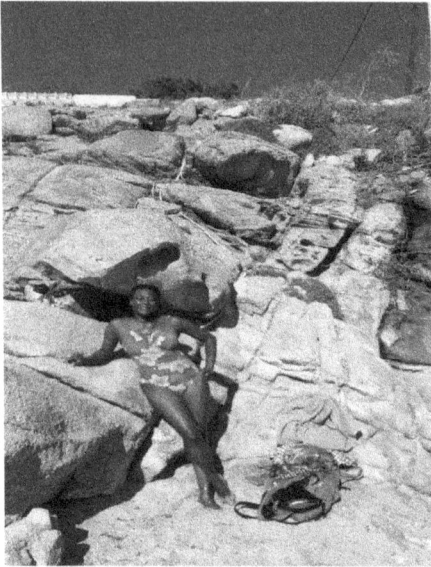

At the beach in Mykonos, Greece, July 2019

October 10, 2019 was officially ten years since God smiled on me and gifted me with a new kidney. I look forward to the many more adventures ahead of me and living my best life. I will continue to trust in Him and treasure each precious day, always remembering, "I can do all things through Christ, who strengthens me." Philippians 4:13.

ACKNOWLEDGEMENTS

I must say a special thank you to Rafael, my dear friend and champion who tirelessly reviewed multiple revisions of this book and offered insightful suggestions that have improved it immensely. I will ever be thankful for your patience and incredible support. God Bless.

I also want to thank all the family, friends, colleagues, mentors, acquaintances, hospital staff, and nurses who may not be included in this book, but who played an important part in my journey. Your support and kindness are deeply valued.

Finally, Dr. Osman and Dr. Geetha. Words cannot express. God is truly awesome. He led me to you in the early days of my diagnosis. Your dedication and care from the time of my diagnosis with Vasculitis to now have been immeasurable. I am truly blessed to have you both in my corner as I continue the fight. Thank you.

www.ingramcontent.com/pod-product-compliance
Lightning Source LLC
Chambersburg PA
CBHW051722090426
42738CB00010B/2034